T0053683

WHAT IT MEANS TO BE A Nurse

A CELEBRATION OF THE HUMOR, HEART, AND HEROES OF EVERY HOSPITAL

The Creator of
SNARKYNURSES

ADAMS MEDIA
NEW YORK LONDON TORONTO SYDNEY NEW DELHI

adamsmedia
Adams Media
An Imprint of Simon & Schuster, Inc.
100 Technology Center Drive
Stoughton, MA 02072

Copyright © 2021 by Simon & Schuster, Inc.

All rights reserved, including the right to reproduce this book or portions thereof in any form whatsoever. For information address Adams Media Subsidiary Rights Department, 1230 Avenue of the Americas, New York, NY 10020.

First Adams Media hardcover edition
April 2021

ADAMS MEDIA and colophon are trademarks of Simon & Schuster.

For information about special discounts for bulk purchases, please contact Simon & Schuster Special Sales at 1-866-506-1949 or business@simonandschuster.com.

The Simon & Schuster Speakers Bureau can bring authors to your live event. For more information or to book an event contact the Simon & Schuster Speakers Bureau at 1-866-248-3049 or visit our website at www.simonspeakers.com.

Interior design by Colleen Cunningham, Erin Alexander, Stephanie Hannus, Alaya Howard, Julia Jacintho, Sylvia McArdle, Victor Watch
Interior images © Getty Images; 123RF

Manufactured in the U.S.A.

10 9 8 7 6 5 4 3 2

Library of Congress Cataloging-in-Publication Data
Title: What it means to be a nurse / The creator of snarkynurses.
Description: First Adams Media hardcover edition. | Avon, Massachusetts: Adams Media, 2021. | Series: What it means.
Identifiers: LCCN 2020034988 | ISBN 9781507215340 (hc) | ISBN 9781507215357 (ebook)
Subjects: LCSH: Nursing--Humor. | Nurses--Anecdotes.
Classification: LCC RT61 . W44 2021 | DDC 610.73--dc23
LC record available at https://lccn.loc.gov/2020034988

ISBN 978-1-5072-1534-0
ISBN 978-1-5072-1535-7 (ebook)

Many of the designations used by manufacturers and sellers to distinguish their products are claimed as trademarks. Where those designations appear in this book and Simon & Schuster, Inc., was aware of a trademark claim, the designations have been printed with initial capital letters.

Dedication

To my mom—
thank you for everything, especially for
instilling that twisted sense of humor!

And to my sugar bean—
perhaps someday you will see this and think
your mom was once kind of awesome.

Introduction

Do you hear call lights, IV pumps, and telemetry alarms in your sleep?

Did your patient just get out of bed without assistance for the seventy-seventh time this shift?

Despite the wild, eye-rolling moments, would you still choose nursing time and time again?

If so, you're clearly a nurse!

Nursing is likely one of the biggest loves of your life. You see life, death, and everything in between. While you may have started out choosing nursing as a career, eventually it becomes part of who you ARE. You live for moments when a parent finally holds their baby in their arms, a treatment plan works, or your patient laughs for the first time in literally days…even if it was because you tripped over your own clogs while walking into their room.

These moments and so many more are what make this profession so fulfilling. Nursing isn't all hilariously awesome coworkers and patients who know better than to use their call light excessively, so in those more challenging times, it's important to remember nurses are in this together. That's where *What It Means to Be a Nurse* comes in!

Within these pages you'll find more than 150 entries which are designed to pour some sunshine into your day when you need it the most, but also to make you laugh and say "Remember that one time…" to your nurse friends. Both humorous and inspiring, they serve as a reminder of why you chose nursing and why the nursing world needs YOU!

Now grab your nursing mug (you know you have one), fill it with your favorite caffeinated beverage (or wine), and dive into this celebration of nursing!

There may be days I contemplate a different career, but ultimately,

I KNOW

NURSING IS FOR ME AND I AM FOR NURSING.

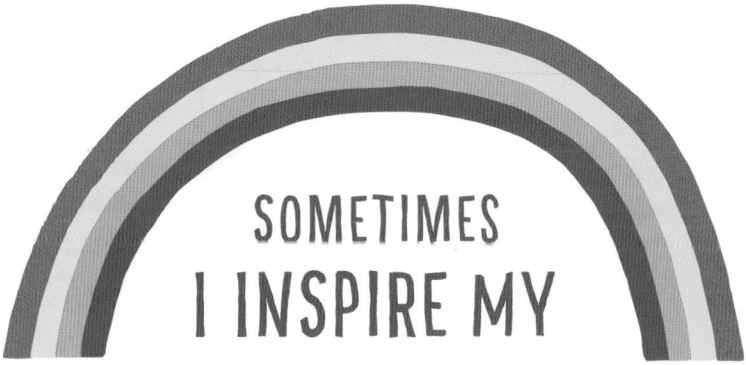

SOMETIMES
I INSPIRE MY
patients;
MORE OFTEN THEY
inspire me.

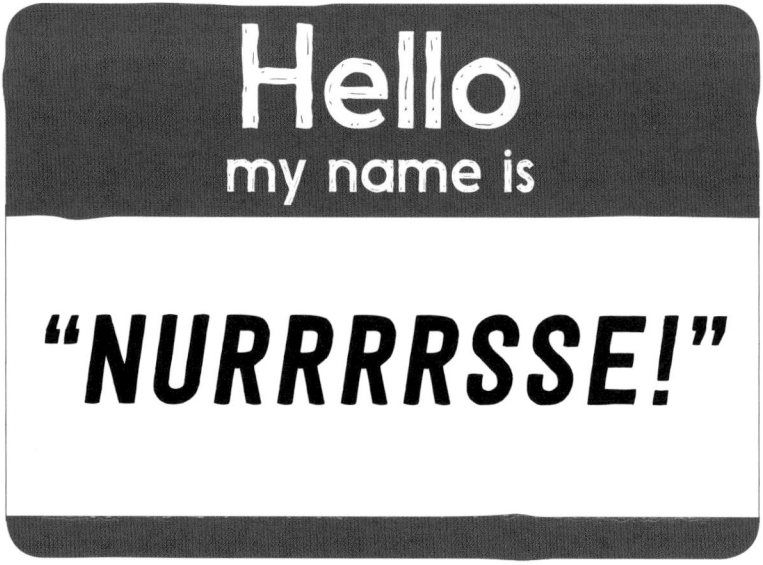
Hello
my name is
"NURRRRSSE!"

Together

WE ALL WORK HARD

for the

BEST

POSSIBLE

OUTCOMES.

YOU MIGHT BE A NURSE IF...
YOU OPEN UP THE DRYER
AND 17 ALCOHOL SWABS
AND TWO OF YOUR
FAVORITE PENS
FALL OUT.

THE THINGS YOU ARE *passionate* ABOUT ARE NOT RANDOM, *they are your calling.*

—FABIENNE FREDRICKSON, FOUNDER OF BOLDHEART

Three words every nurse loves hearing during a coworker's report:

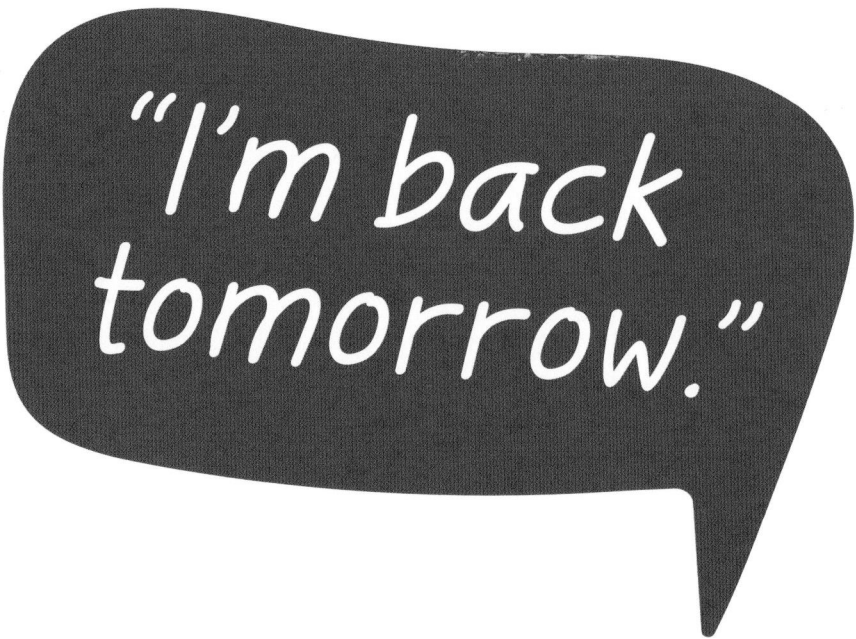

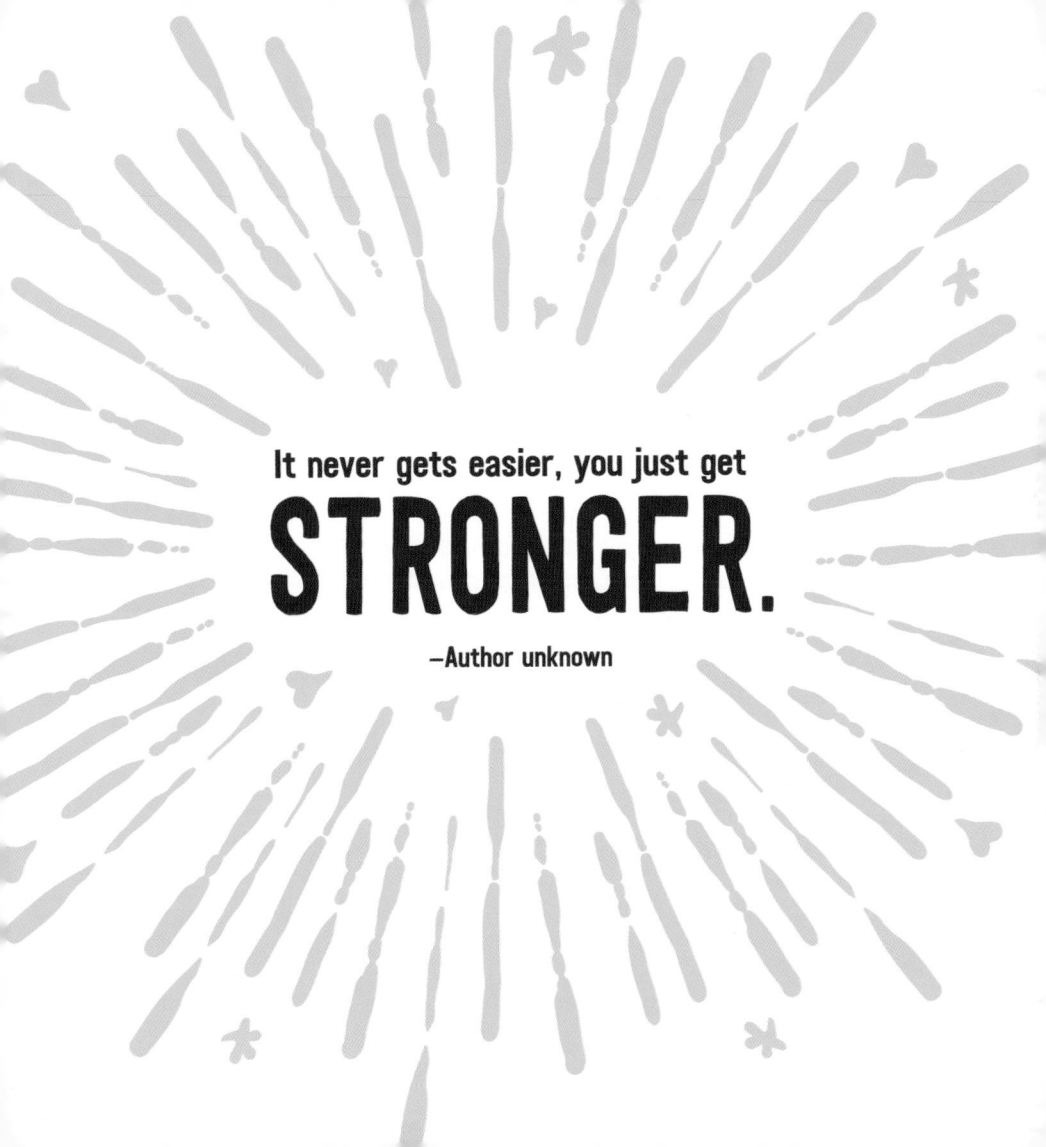
It never gets easier, you just get
STRONGER.
—Author unknown

ADVOCACY

the #1 priority for all nurses.

WHEN YOU'RE A NURSE, YOU KNOW *that* EVERY DAY YOU WILL TOUCH A LIFE *or a* LIFE WILL TOUCH YOURS.

—AUTHOR UNKNOWN

When your manager rolls by and asks how you're doing:

"I'M FINE,
IT'S FINE,
EVERYTHING'S FINE!"

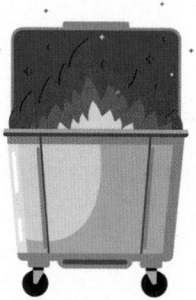

NARRATOR:

"EVERYTHING WAS NOT FINE."

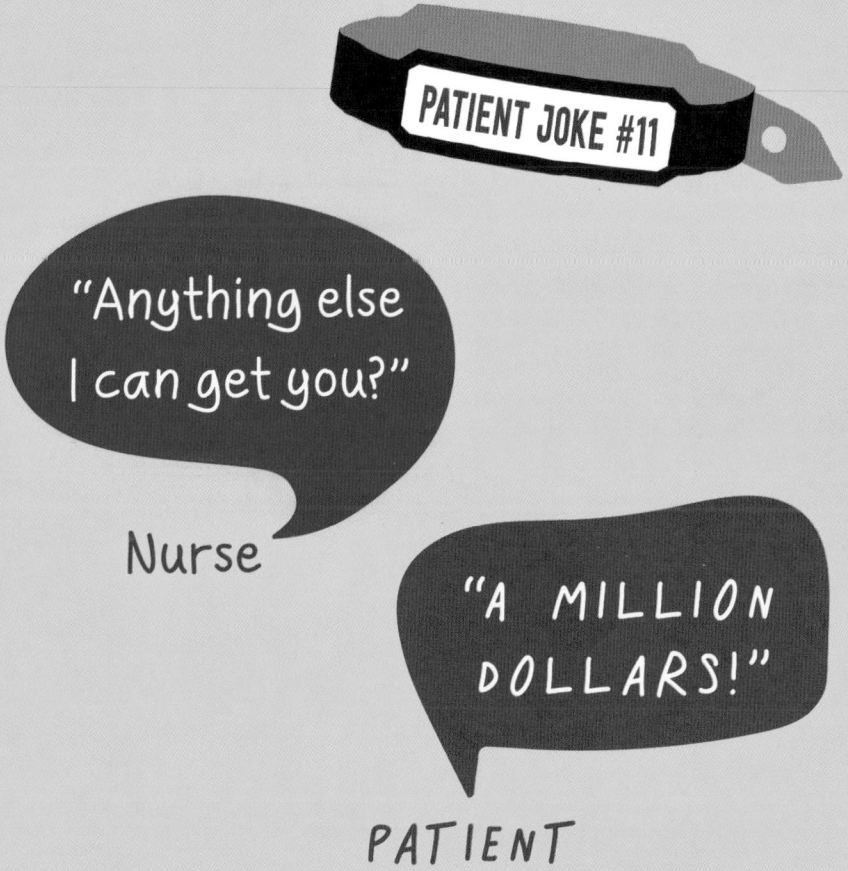
PATIENT JOKE #11
"Anything else I can get you?"
Nurse
"A MILLION DOLLARS!"
PATIENT

STRENGTH

HUMOR

TEAMWORK

COMPASSION

ADVOCATE

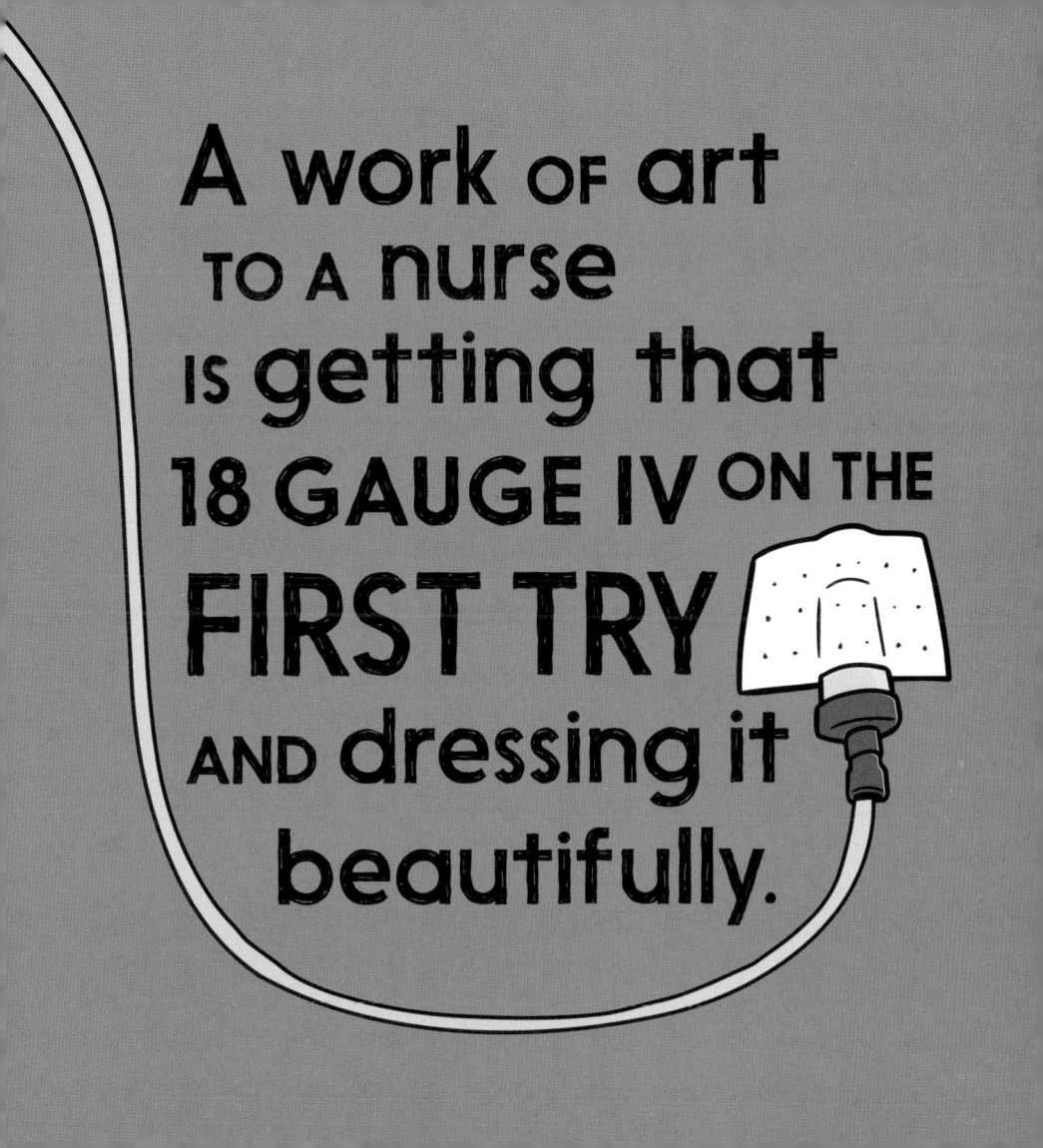
A work OF art
TO A nurse
IS getting that
18 GAUGE IV ON THE
FIRST TRY
AND dressing it
beautifully.

On those really
tough days,
don't forget...

miracles happen.

WHAT INSPIRES A NURSE TO MOVE AT THE SPEED OF LIGHT?

A BED ALARM...

OR FRESH COFFEE IN THE BREAKROOM.

I've learned that people will *forget what you said*, people will *forget what you did*, but

people will never forget *how you made them feel.*

—Maya Angelou, poet

And the winner for least favorite phrase in the hospital is:

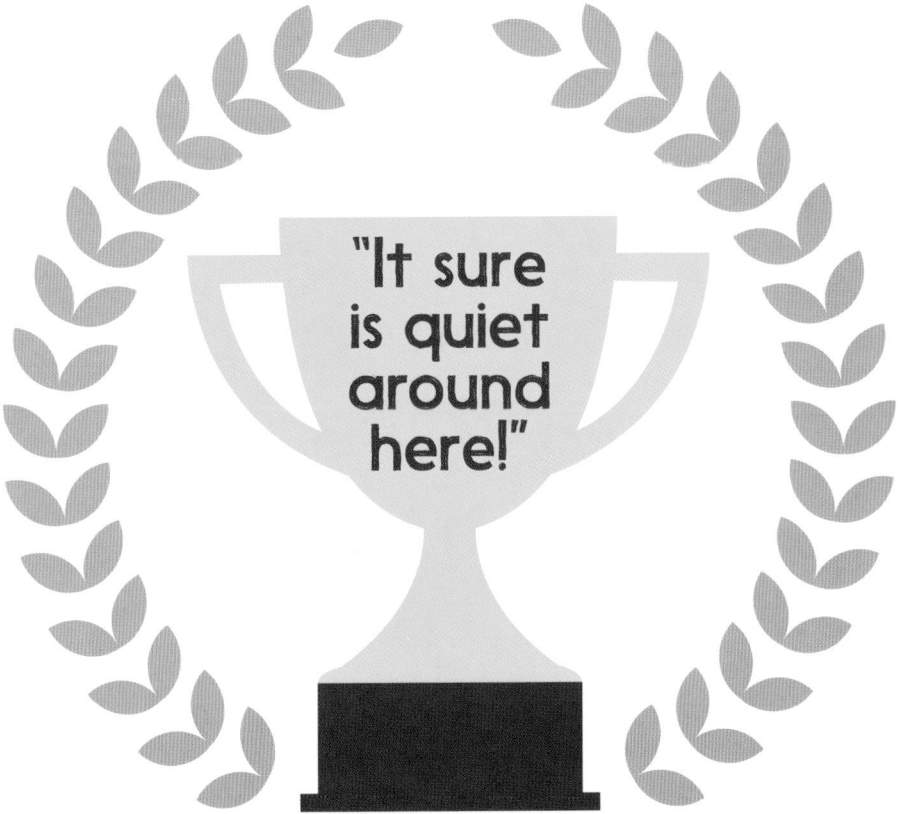

MURPHY'S LAW OF NURSING

#25

AS SOON AS YOU HAVE GOWNED, GLOVED, MASKED, AND WALKED INTO YOUR PATIENT'S ROOM, YOU'LL REMEMBER THREE OTHER THINGS YOU NEEDED TO GET.

THE *best way* TO
find yourself
IS TO
lose yourself
IN THE service
of others.

—MAHATMA GANDHI,
lawyer, politician, and social activist

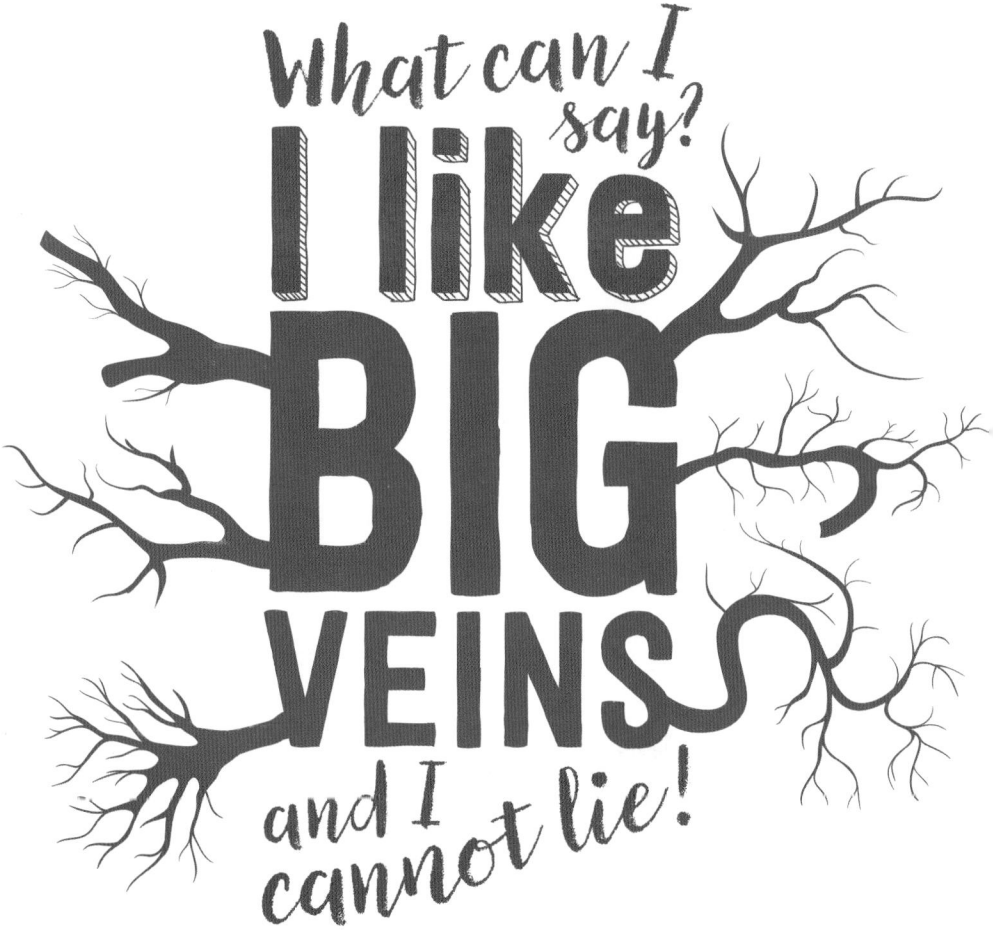
What can I say?
I like
BIG
VEINS
and I cannot lie!

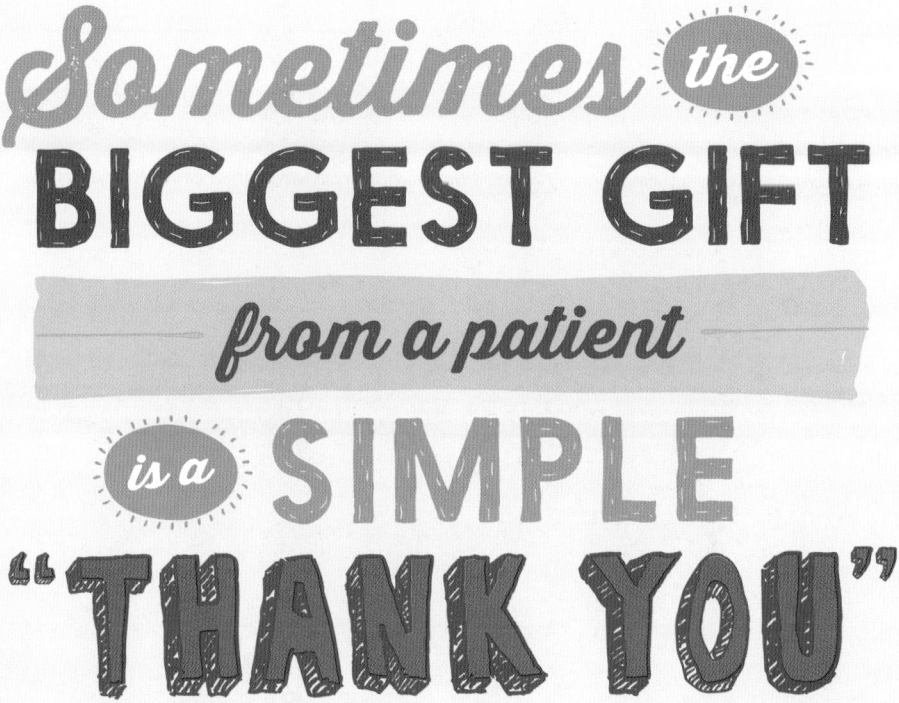
Sometimes the
BIGGEST GIFT
from a patient
is a SIMPLE
"THANK YOU"

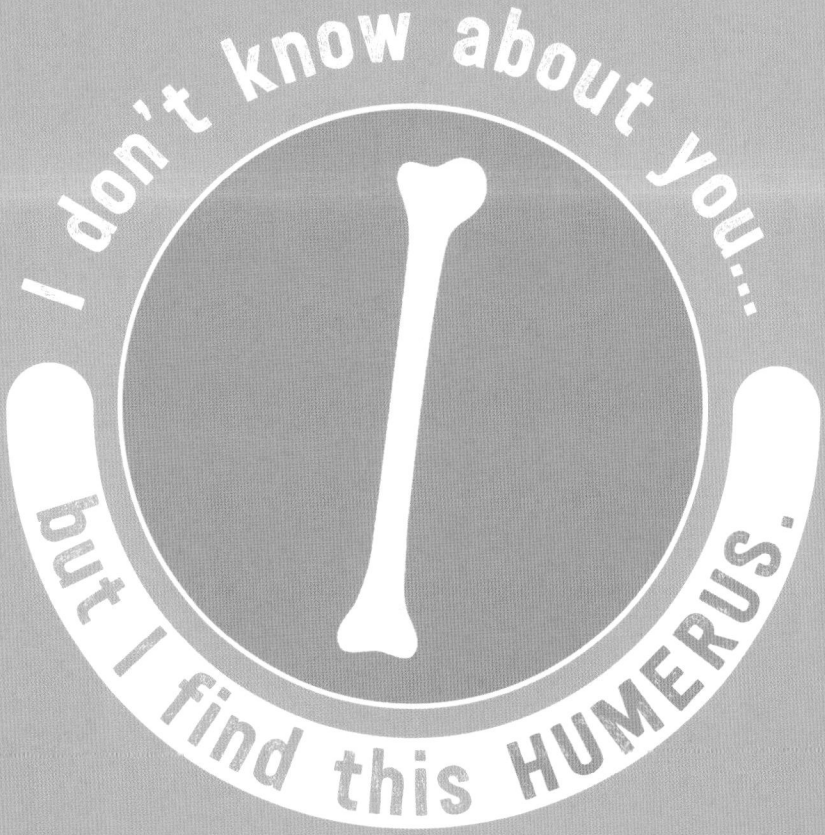
I don't know about you...
but I find this HUMERUS.

It doesn't *matter*
WHO you are,
I will *take care*
of YOU with
a *devoted* ♥

My best friend's name is Pam.
She's pretty low-key and great to be around.

Lorazepam.

Diazepam.

Clonazepam.

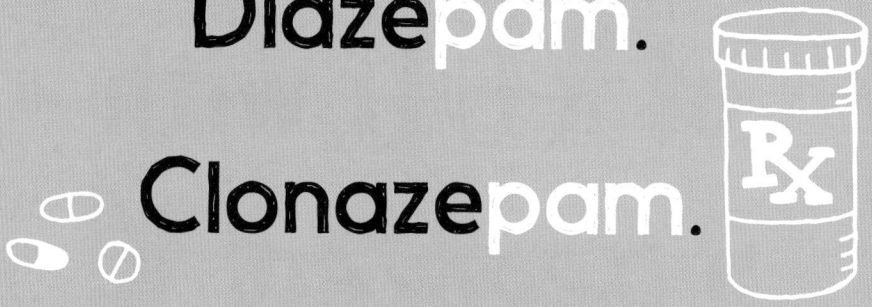

"A hero is an ordinary individual who finds the **STRENGTH** to **PERSEVERE** and **ENDURE** in spite of overwhelming obstacles."

—Christopher Reeve, actor

SOME OF THE
best friends
YOU WILL HAVE
ARE YOUR
coworkers.

THERE ARE NO
FRIENDSHIPS LIKE
nurse
friendships.

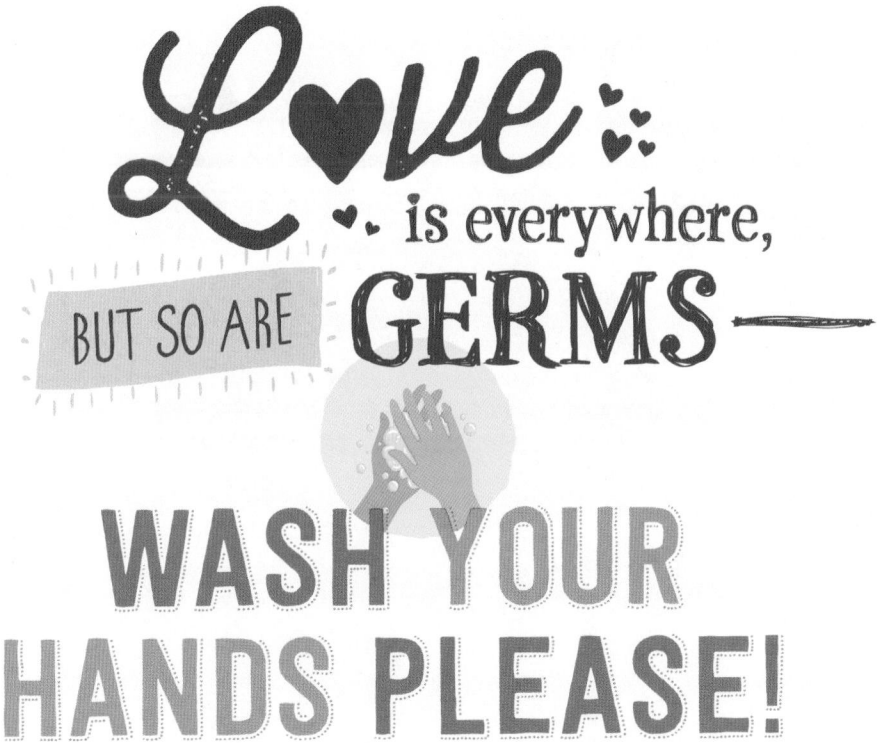
Love is everywhere,
BUT SO ARE GERMS —
WASH YOUR HANDS PLEASE!

NURSING

is a career where you

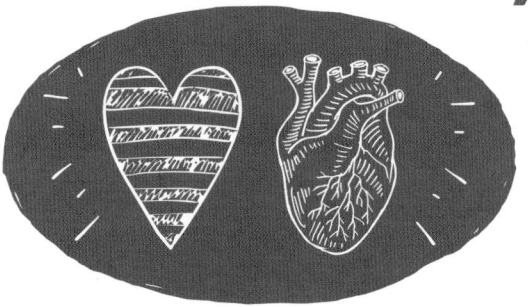

understand both

HEARTS.

NURSES...
SINGLE-HANDEDLY
KEEPING THE
ECONOMY AFLOAT
BY BUYING
CUTE SCRUBS
AND BADGE REELS.

I'M NOT TELLING YOU
IT'S GOING TO BE *easy.*
I'M TELLING YOU
IT'S GOING TO BE
worth it.

—Art Williams, insurance executive

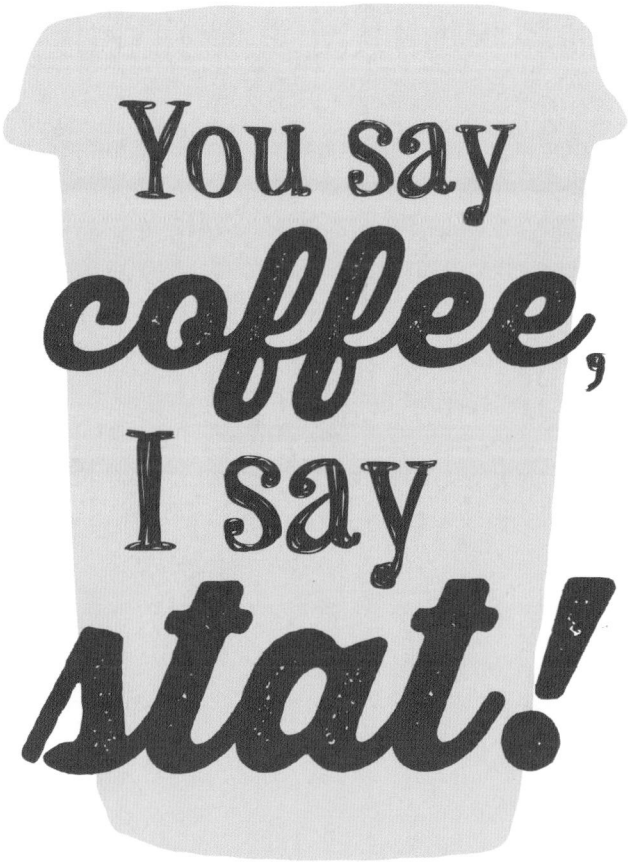
You say
coffee,
I say
stat!

YOU MIGHT BE A NURSE IF...

YOU SURVIVED A 12-HOUR SHIFT ON *graham crackers* AND *ginger ale* FROM THE NUTRITION ROOM

MURPHY'S LAW OF NURSING

WHENEVER YOU FINALLY HAVE TIME TO PEE, EVERY BATHROOM WILL BE OCCUPIED.

Nursing hide-and-seek:

searching for a

LITTLE WHITE PILL

among the bedsheets.

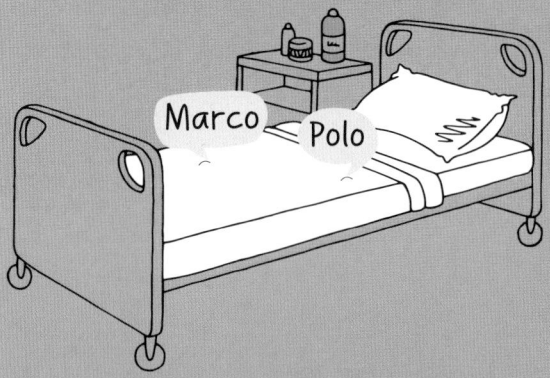

Just when you think
you've got it all together...

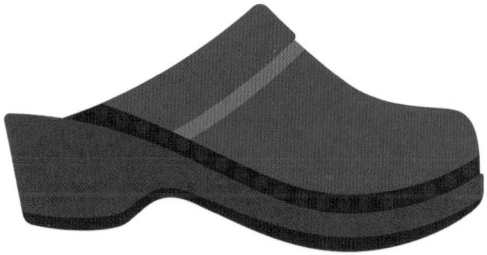

you trip and almost break
a cankle in your clogs.

Wait...who is Don Gloves?

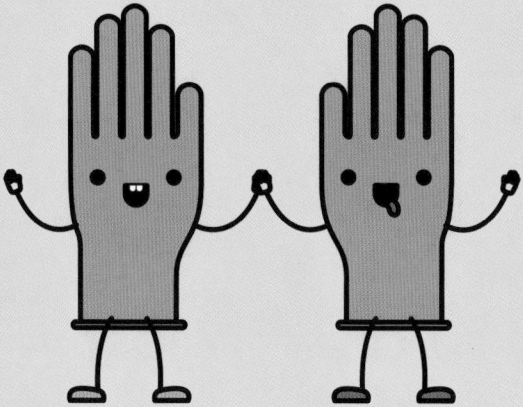

Sometimes when the going gets TOUGH, ya just gotta go with the Flo.

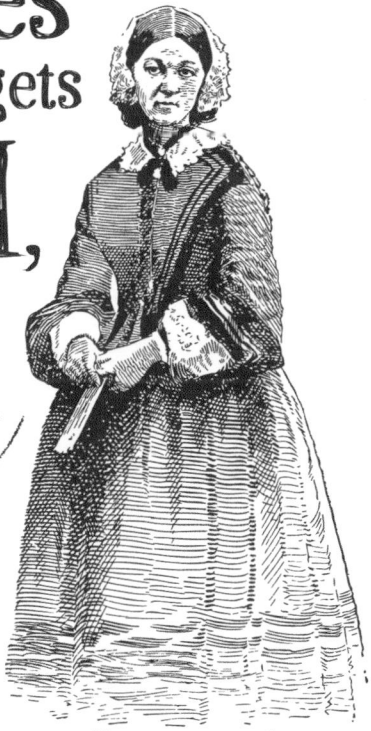

Florence Nightingale

EIGHT TIMES OUT OF TEN I ASK MY PATIENT WHAT DAY IT IS AND DON'T EVEN KNOW THE ANSWER MYSELF.

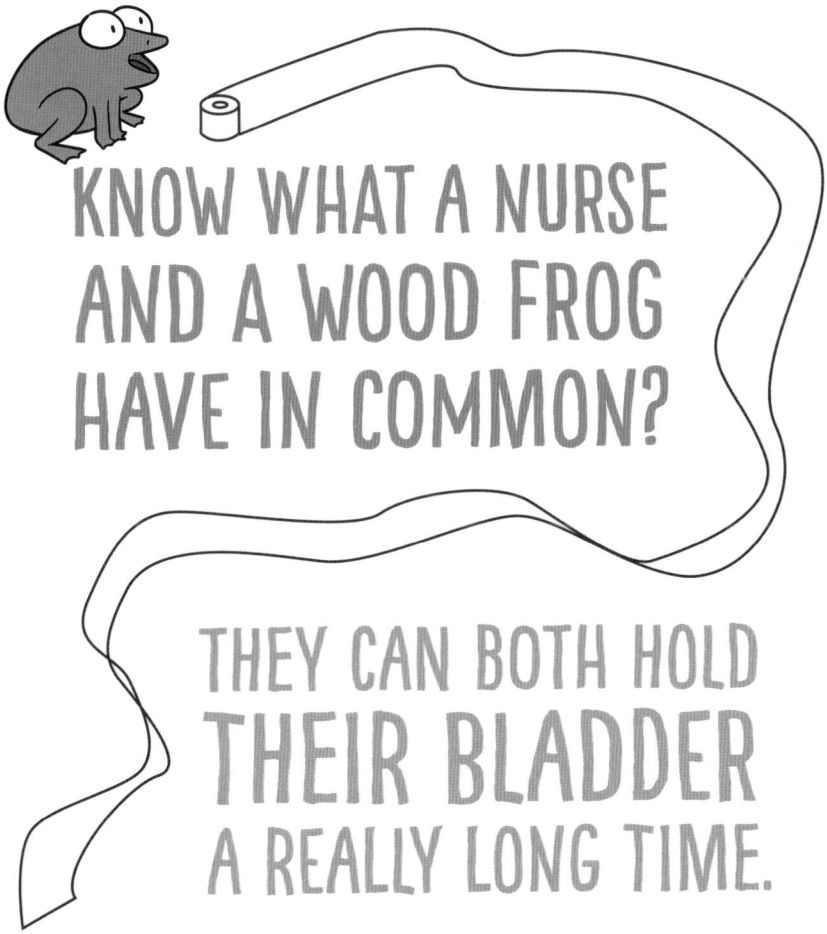
KNOW WHAT A NURSE AND A WOOD FROG HAVE IN COMMON?
THEY CAN BOTH HOLD THEIR BLADDER A REALLY LONG TIME.

It only takes one
kind, thankful,
and fun-loving
patient to erase
so many hard days.

Nothing beats the satisfaction of taking off your

compression socks

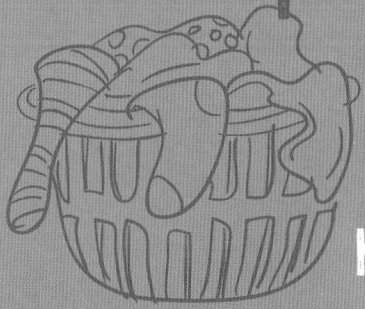

after twelve hours of pounding the hospital pavement.

YOU MIGHT BE A NURSE IF...

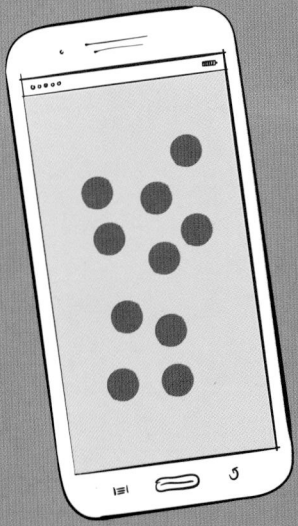

YOU'VE RECEIVED TEXTS FROM FRIENDS AND FAMILY
ASKING YOU TO EXAMINE A RASH.

Are you even a nurse if you haven't heard **CALL LIGHTS** going off in your sleep?

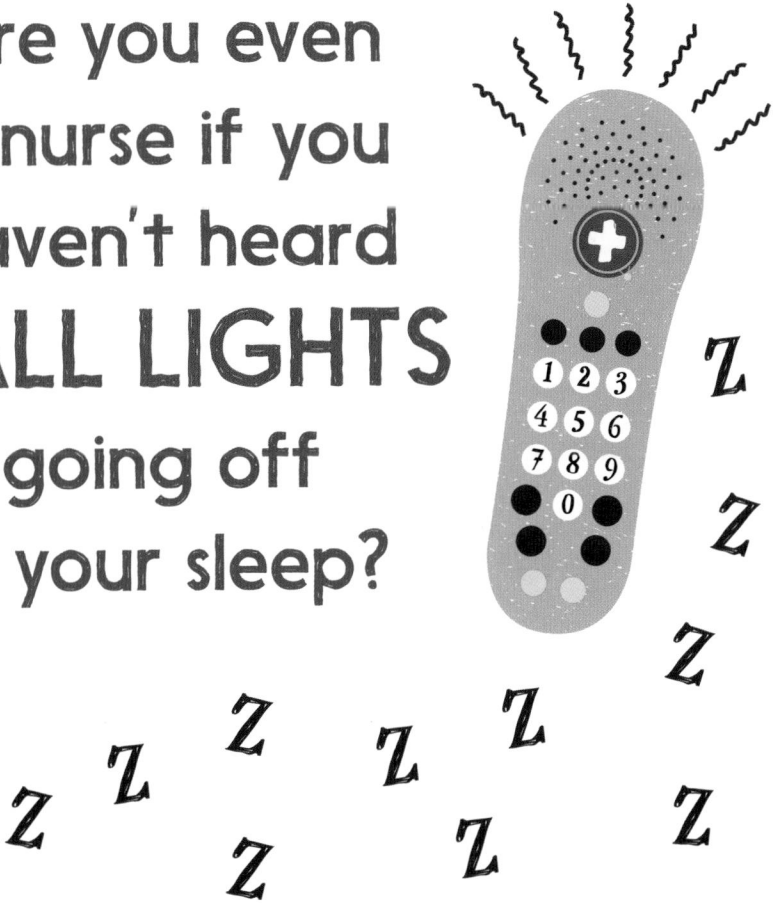

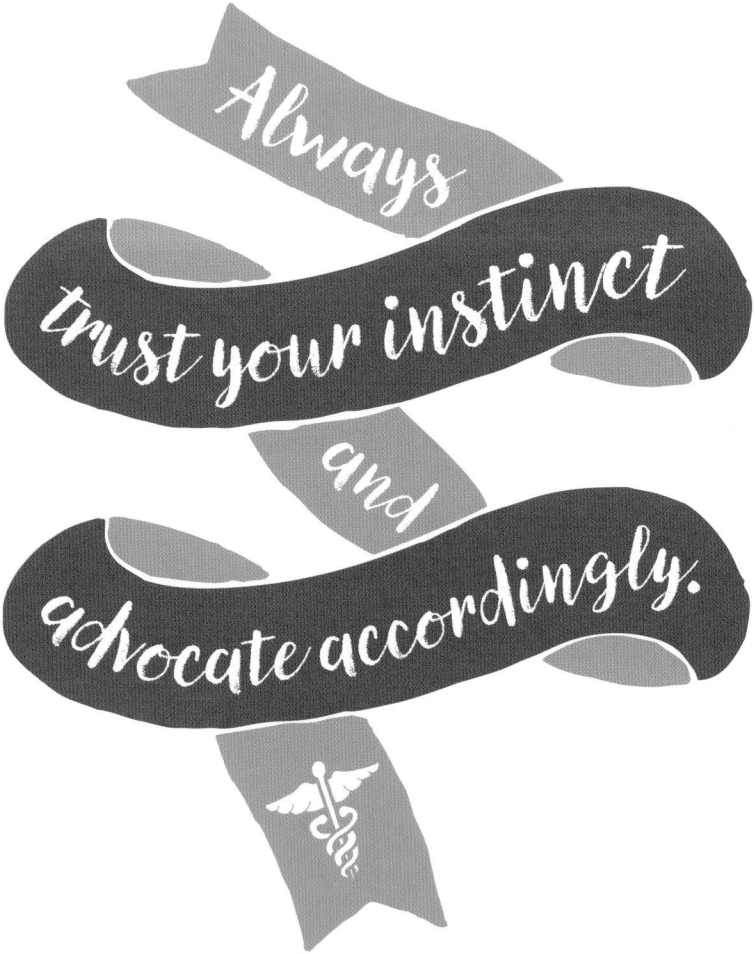
Always
trust your instinct
and
advocate accordingly.

I ALWAYS TELL MY PATIENTS:

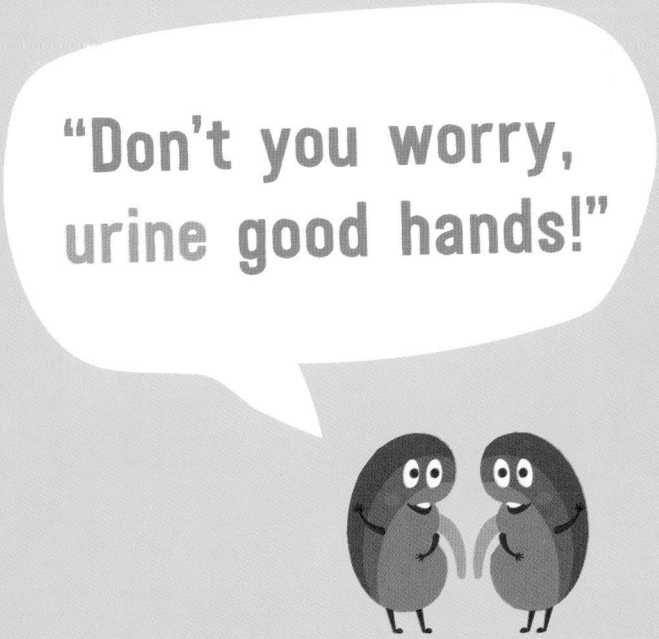

SIZE *does* MATTER!

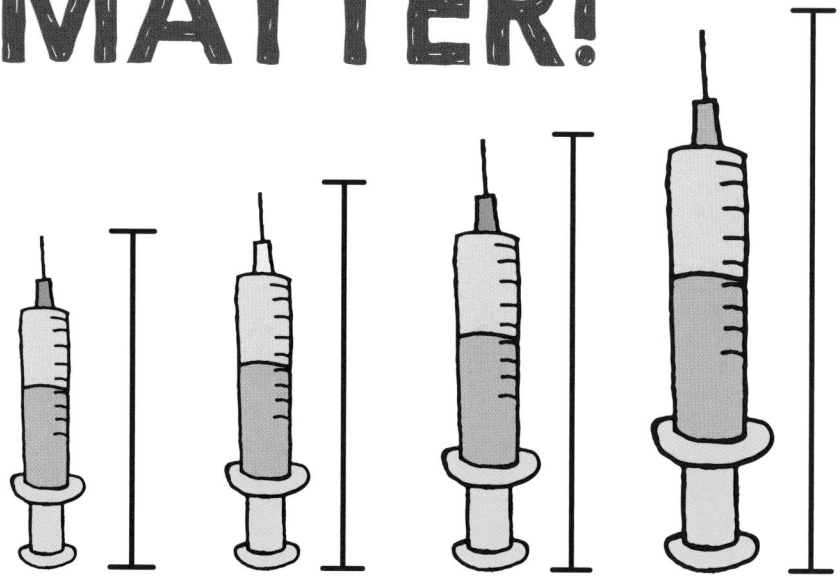

TO ERR IS HUMAN.

Every nurse has made a mistake; it's about how you *move forward* and *improve your practice* from there.

NURSES

ASSESS, advocate,
educate, encourage,
inspire, empathize,
LEAD, respect,
and *innovate*.

Know what day it is?

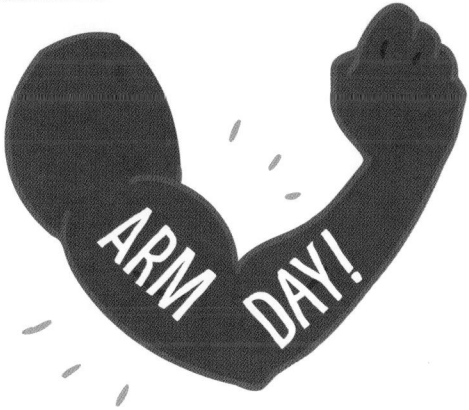

TWO SETS of reconstituting piperacillin-tazobactam, THREE SETS overhead IV fluid lifts, and INFINITE SETS of turning, lifting, and boosting patients.

Oh hey there...

I know you're super busy and all, but...

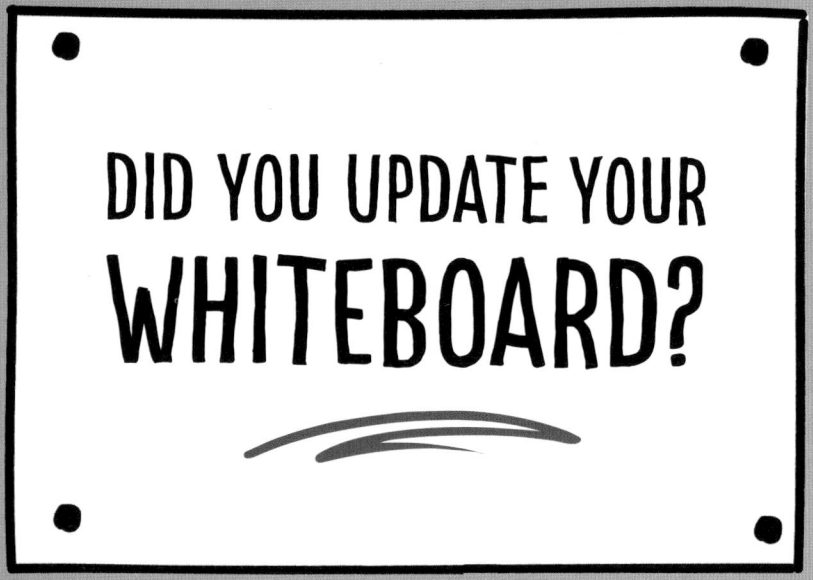

SOMETHING YOU CAN ALWAYS COUNT ON...

the pharmacy

WILL BE REFILLING MEDICATIONS WHEN YOU NEED A MED

STAT.

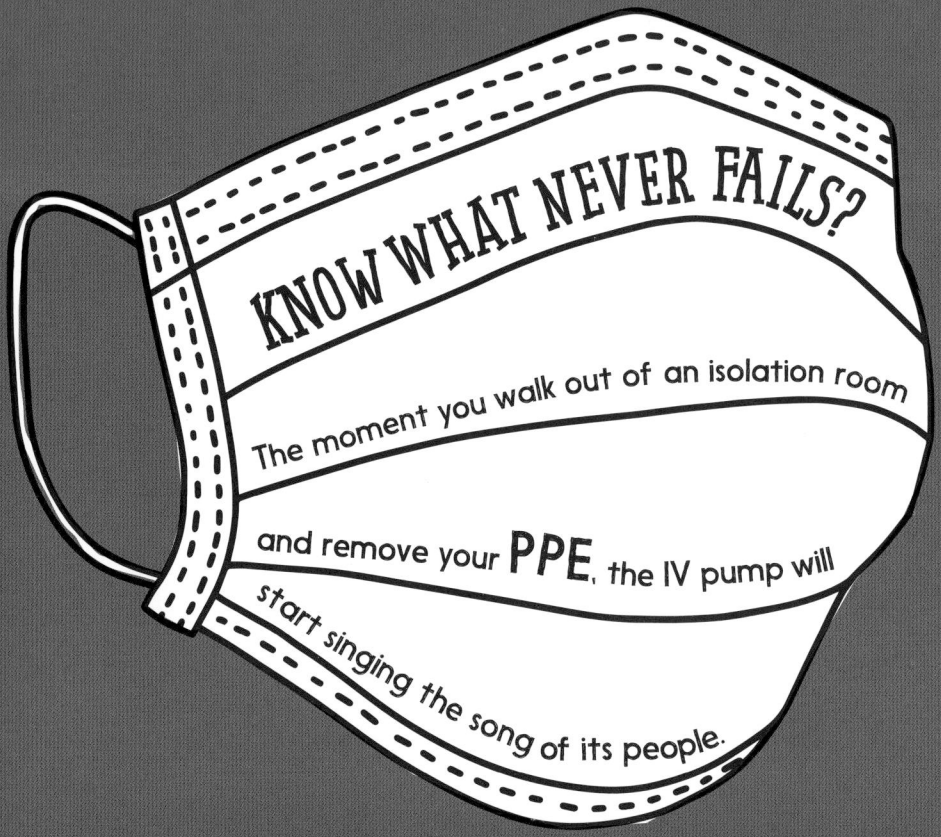
KNOW WHAT NEVER FAILS?
The moment you walk out of an isolation room
and remove your PPE, the IV pump will
start singing the song of its people.

Even if you don't think
you made a difference,

YOU DID.

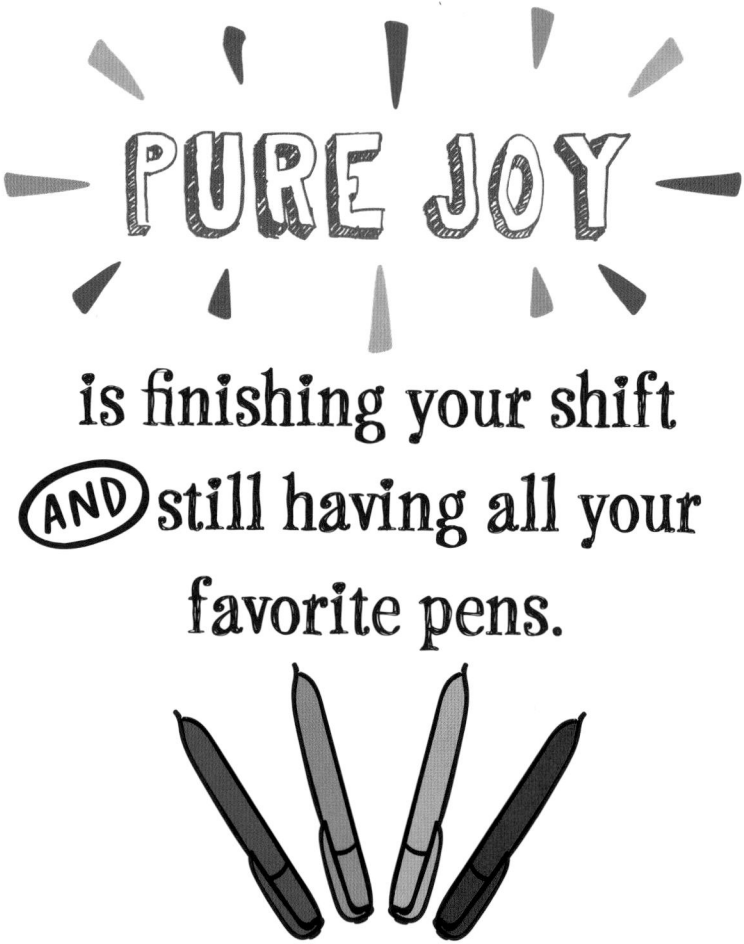
PURE JOY
is finishing your shift
AND still having all your
favorite pens.

Nothing is more

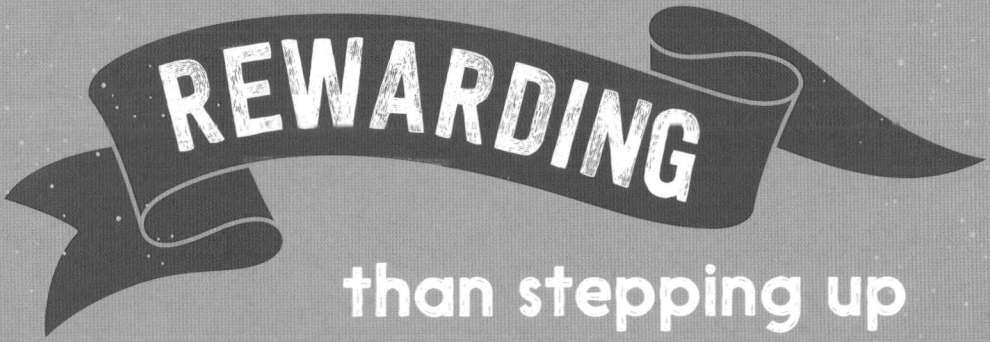

than stepping up to advocate for your patient when they are unable to do it themselves.

I'm sorry, I can't because:

A

I'm on call.

B

I work tomorrow.

C

I'd rather sleep.

D

I have to go to my brother's best friend's hamster's funeral.

Telemetry:

where you can tell if your patient is up to no good

SIMPLY BY THEIR EKG TRACING.

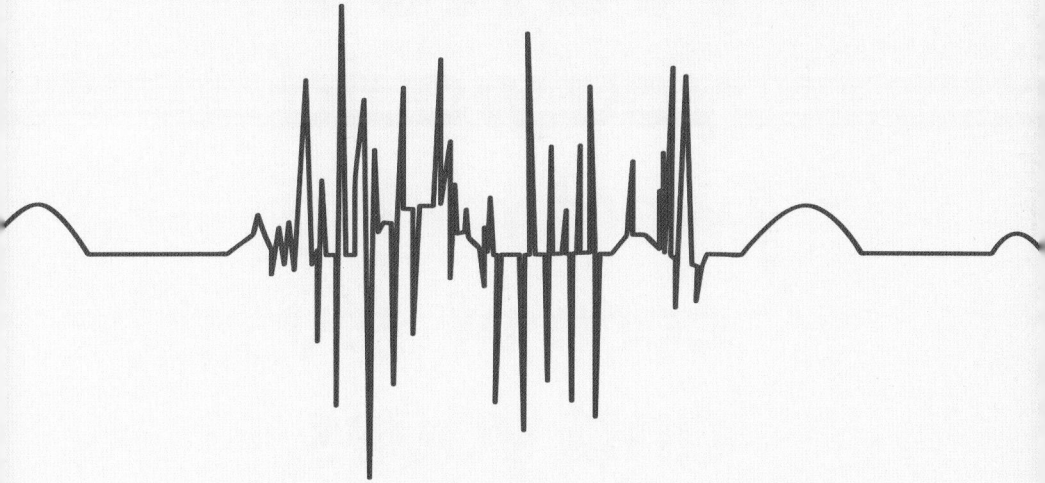

Strive to be
the kind of
NURSE
you would
want taking
care of you
and yours.

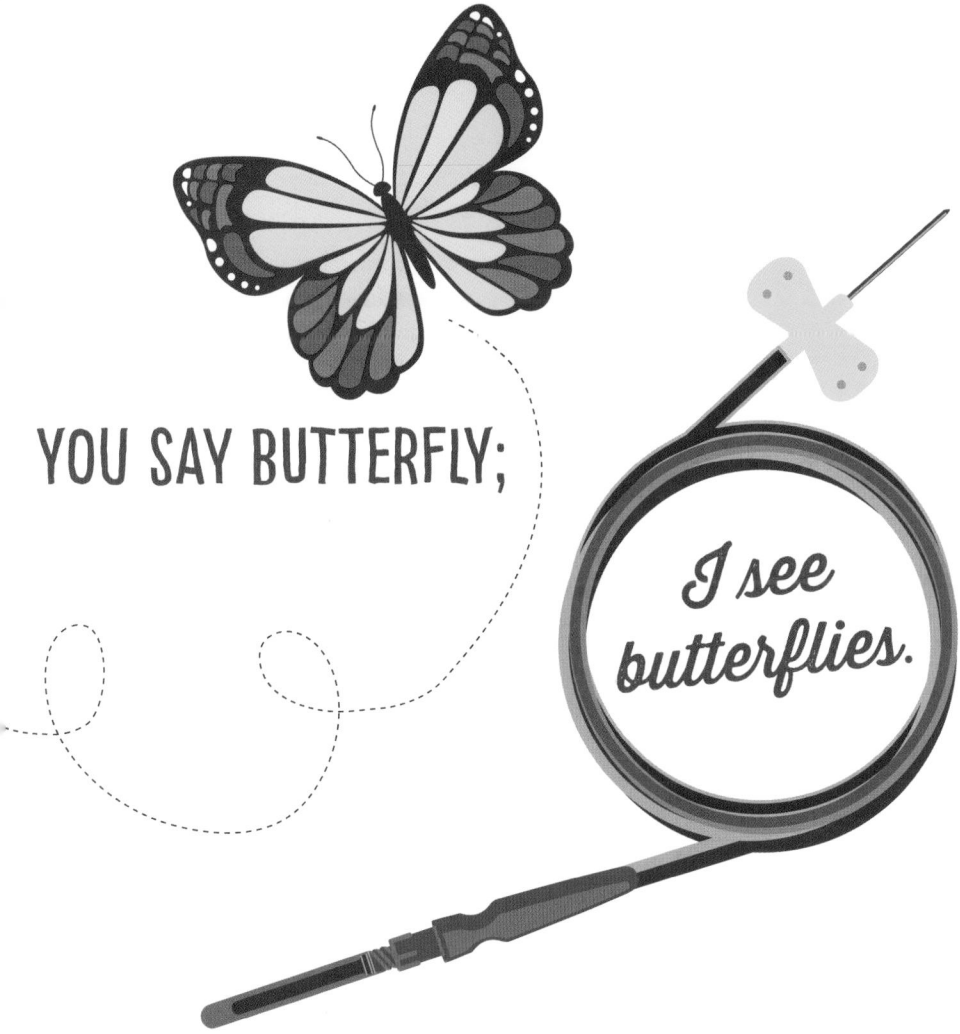
YOU SAY BUTTERFLY;
I see butterflies.

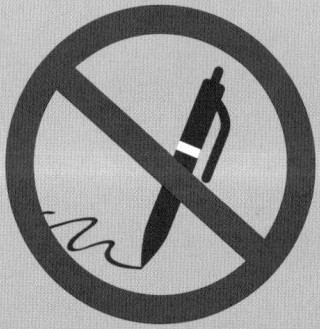

Nurses may share tips and tricks to make your shift easier but don't ask to borrow their pen.

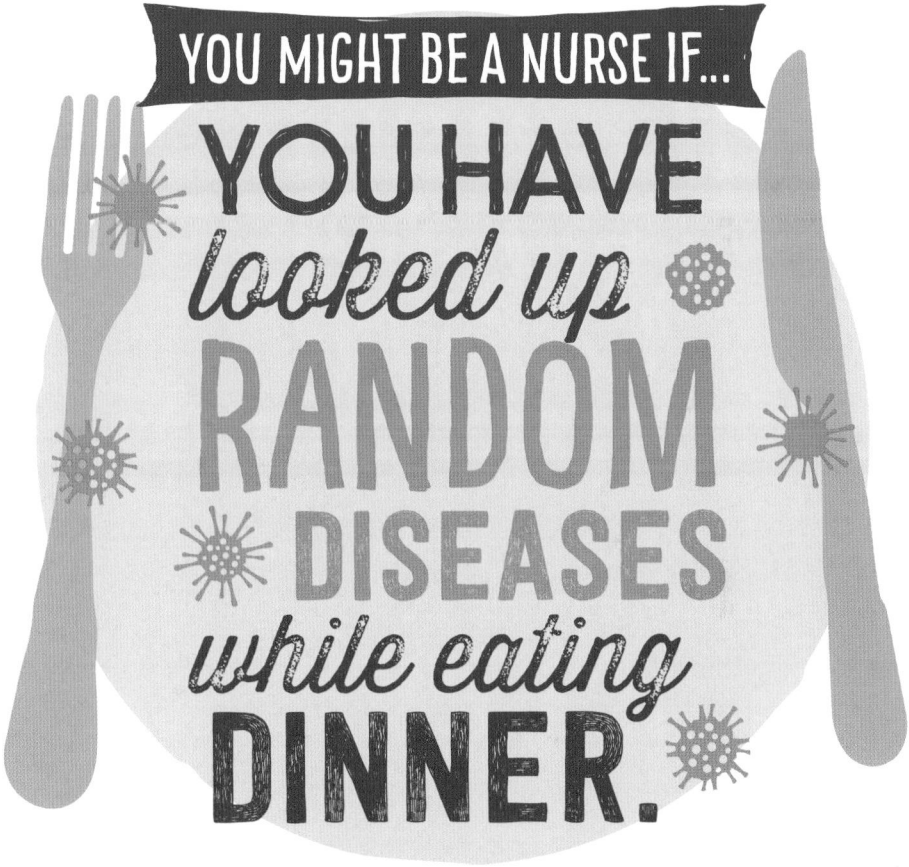
YOU MIGHT BE A NURSE IF...
YOU HAVE
looked up
RANDOM
DISEASES
while eating
DINNER.

The magic of nursing lies in the little things:

Seeing your patient succeed.

Mastering a skill that you've struggled with.

Making lifelong friends.

Laughing about the absurdity of this profession.

A NURSE'S MEMORY IN A NUTSHELL:

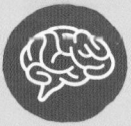

You'll remember your patient's entire medical history but get to the supply room and forget four of the five things you needed.

True

NURSING **MAGIC**

IS

WHEN YOU CAN MAKE A

patient laugh

DESPITE THEIR CURRENT SITUATION.

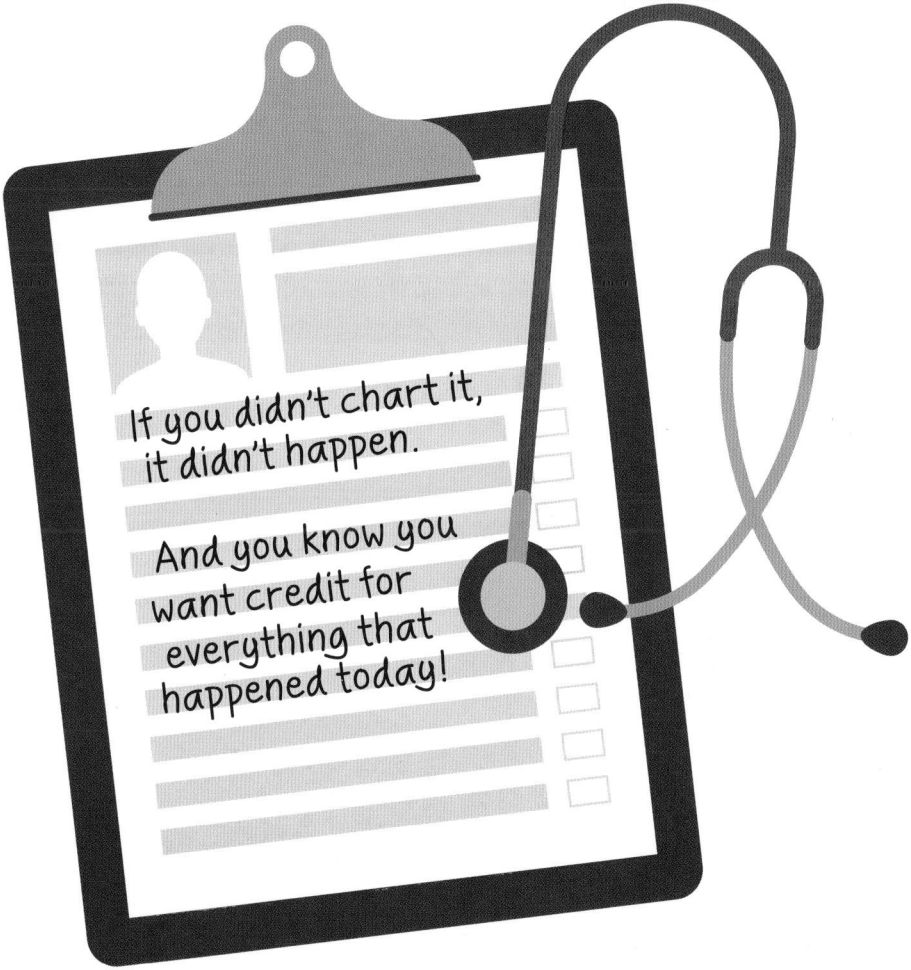
If you didn't chart it,
it didn't happen.
And you know you
want credit for
everything that
happened today!

» NEVER »

UNDERESTIMATE

YOUR ABILITY TO

help a patient feel safe

AND

well taken care of.

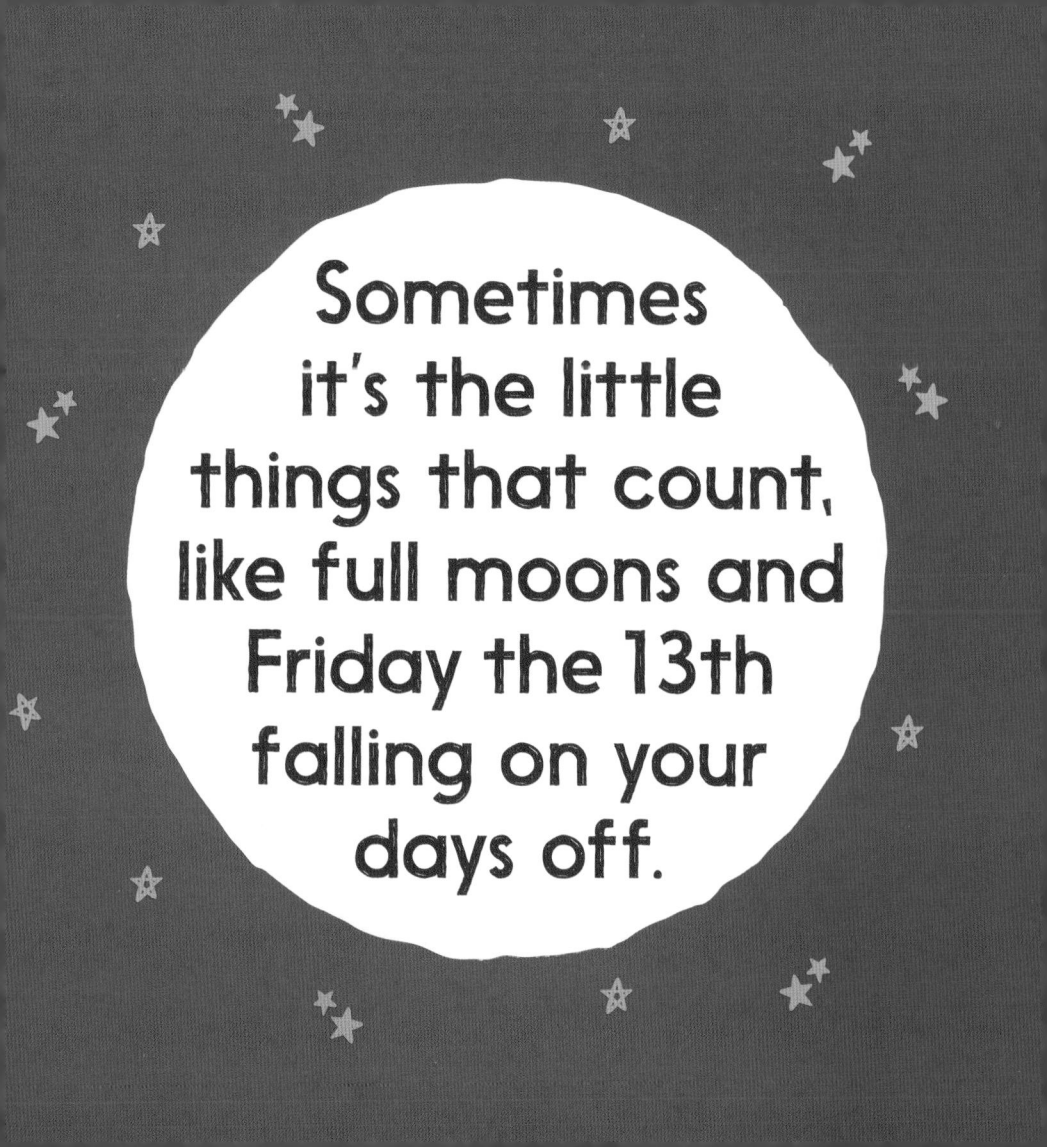
Sometimes
it's the little
things that count,
like full moons and
Friday the 13th
falling on your
days off.

RAISE YOUR HAND

IF YOU'VE EVER WANTED

TO THROW

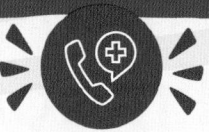

a call light

OUT THE

WINDOW.

MAY YOU ALWAYS HAVE THE

enthusiasm OF

A NEW GRAD NURSE

AND THE

HUMOR,

wisdom, and

UNFLAPPABLE

PRESENCE OF

A 30-YEAR NURSE.

You know what they say:

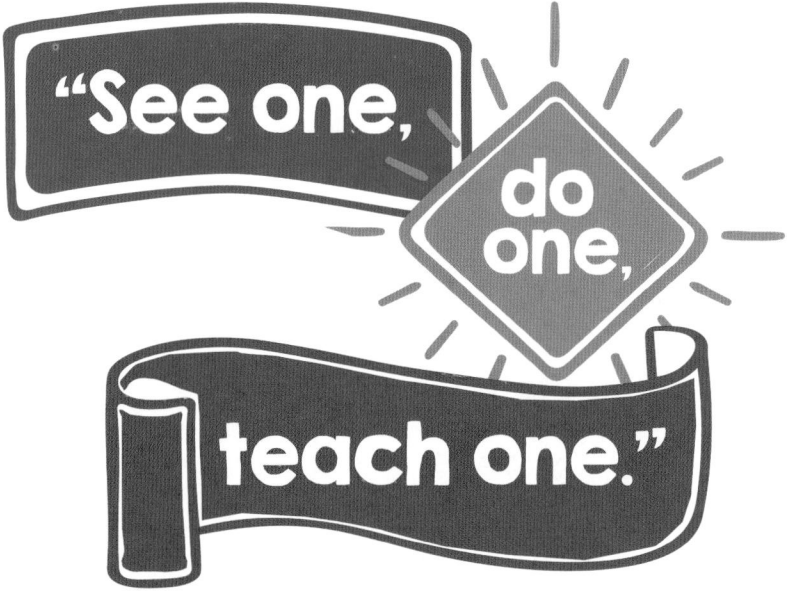

SOMETIMES YOU JUST NEED A PILE OF

doughnuts

TO SHOW UP ON THE BREAKROOM TABLE.

have you tried turning it off and on again?

Love,
adenosine

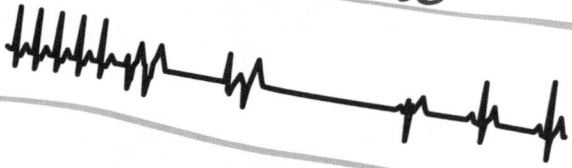

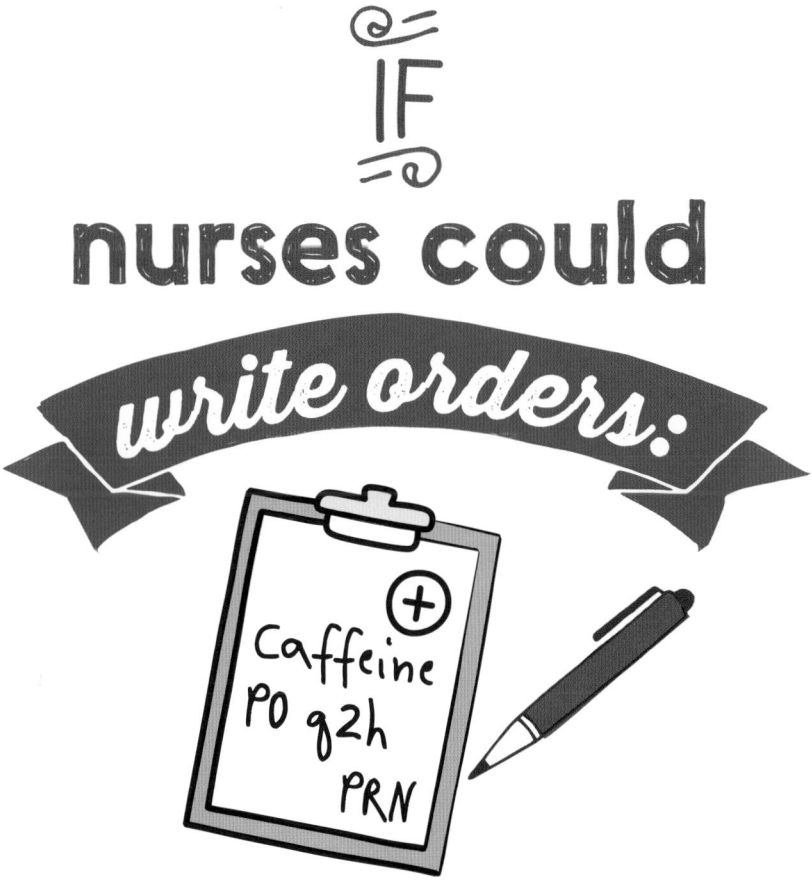
IF
nurses could
write orders:
Caffeine
PO q2h
PRN

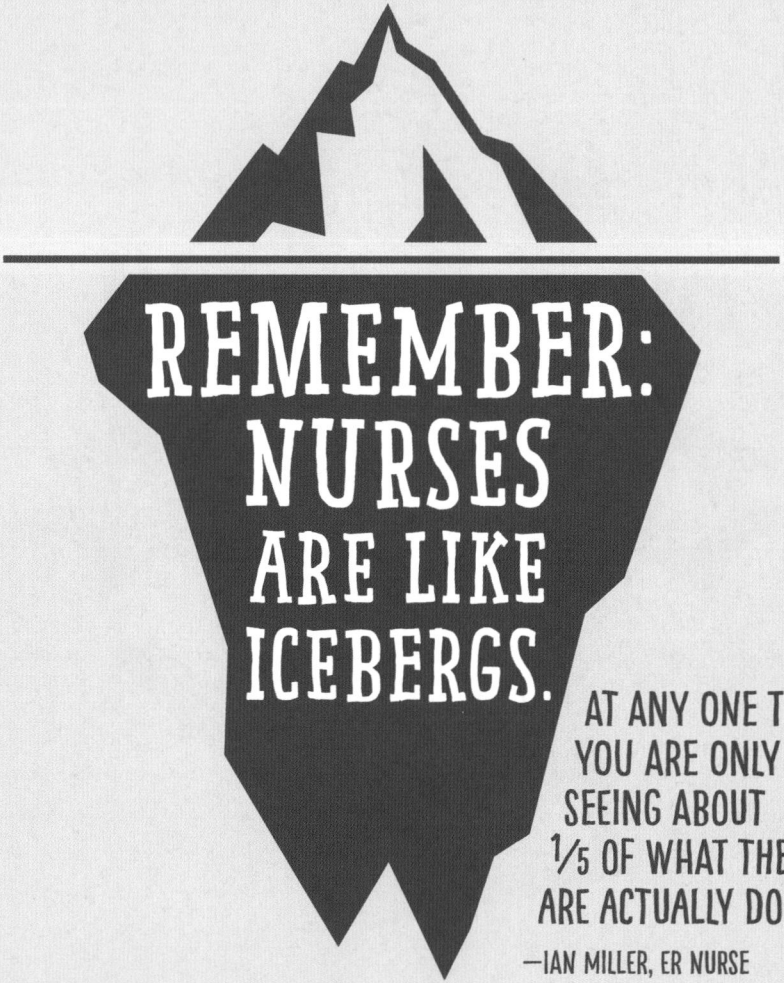
REMEMBER:
NURSES
ARE LIKE
ICEBERGS.
AT ANY ONE TIME,
YOU ARE ONLY
SEEING ABOUT
1/5 OF WHAT THEY
ARE ACTUALLY DOING.
—IAN MILLER, ER NURSE

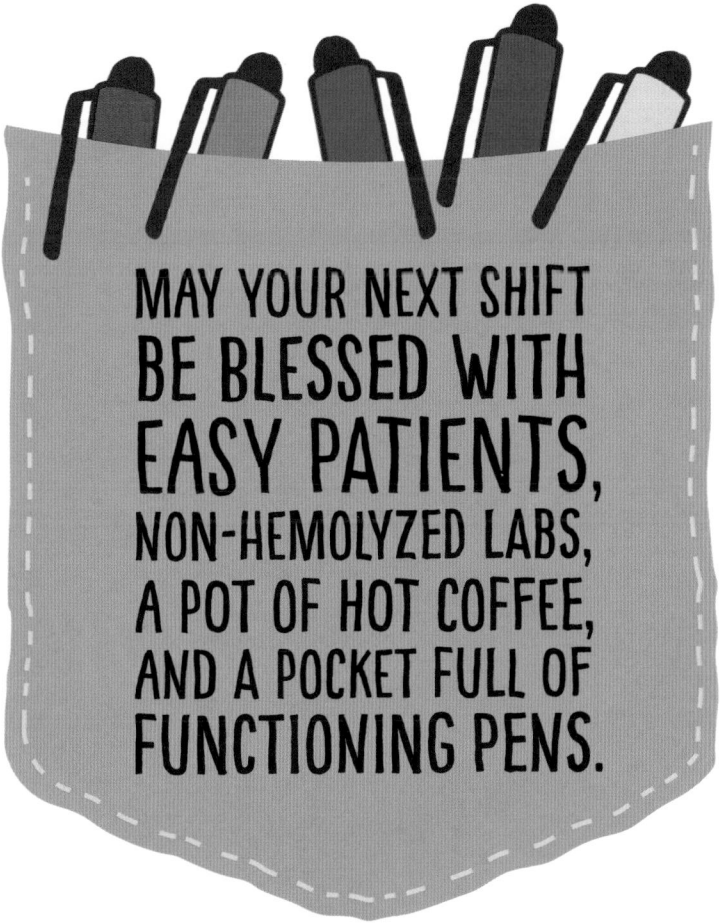
MAY YOUR NEXT SHIFT
BE BLESSED WITH
EASY PATIENTS,
NON-HEMOLYZED LABS,
A POT OF HOT COFFEE,
AND A POCKET FULL OF
FUNCTIONING PENS.

TINY BLESSINGS #117

When you see
a ventricular tachycardia
alarm and run in to find
your patient brushing
their teeth!

When I think about all the patients and their loved ones I have worked with over the years, I know most of them don't remember me, nor I them. But I do know that I gave a little piece of myself to each of them, and they to me, and those threads make up the tapestry that is my career in nursing.

—Donna Wilk Cardillo, RN and author

No one understands the frustration of an IV pump

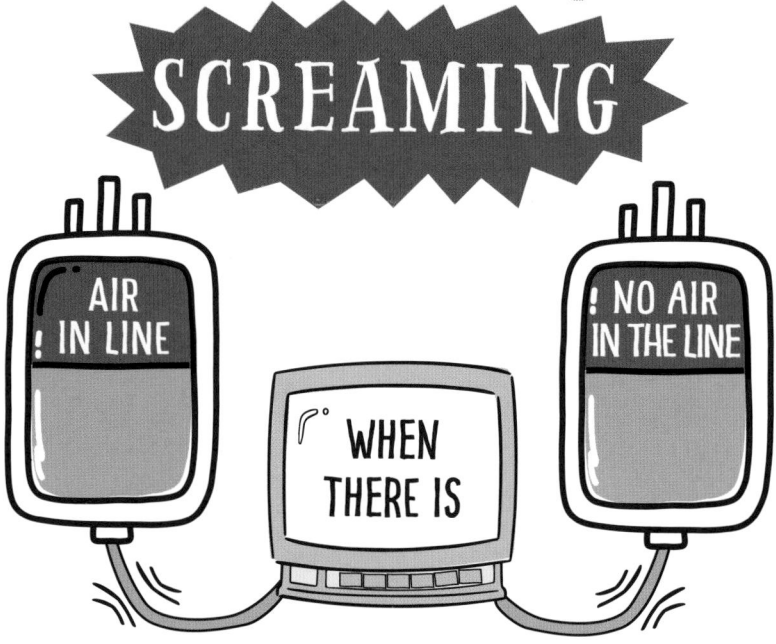

MOST NURSES WILL GIVE *medical advice*

FOR TACOS

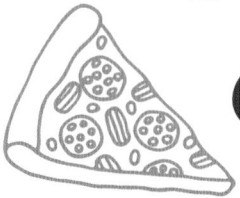

OR PIZZA

OR ...WINE!

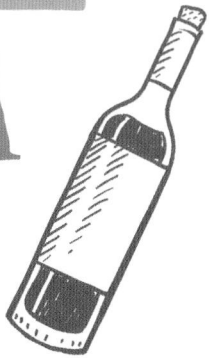

Friendly reminder:

Unless there's an emergency,

NO RUNNING

&

NO YELLING

RAISE YOUR HAND
IF YOU'VE EVER FELT

PERSONALLY

VICTIMIZED

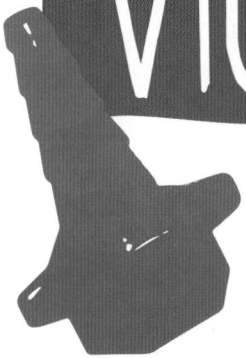

BY A CHRISTMAS
TREE.

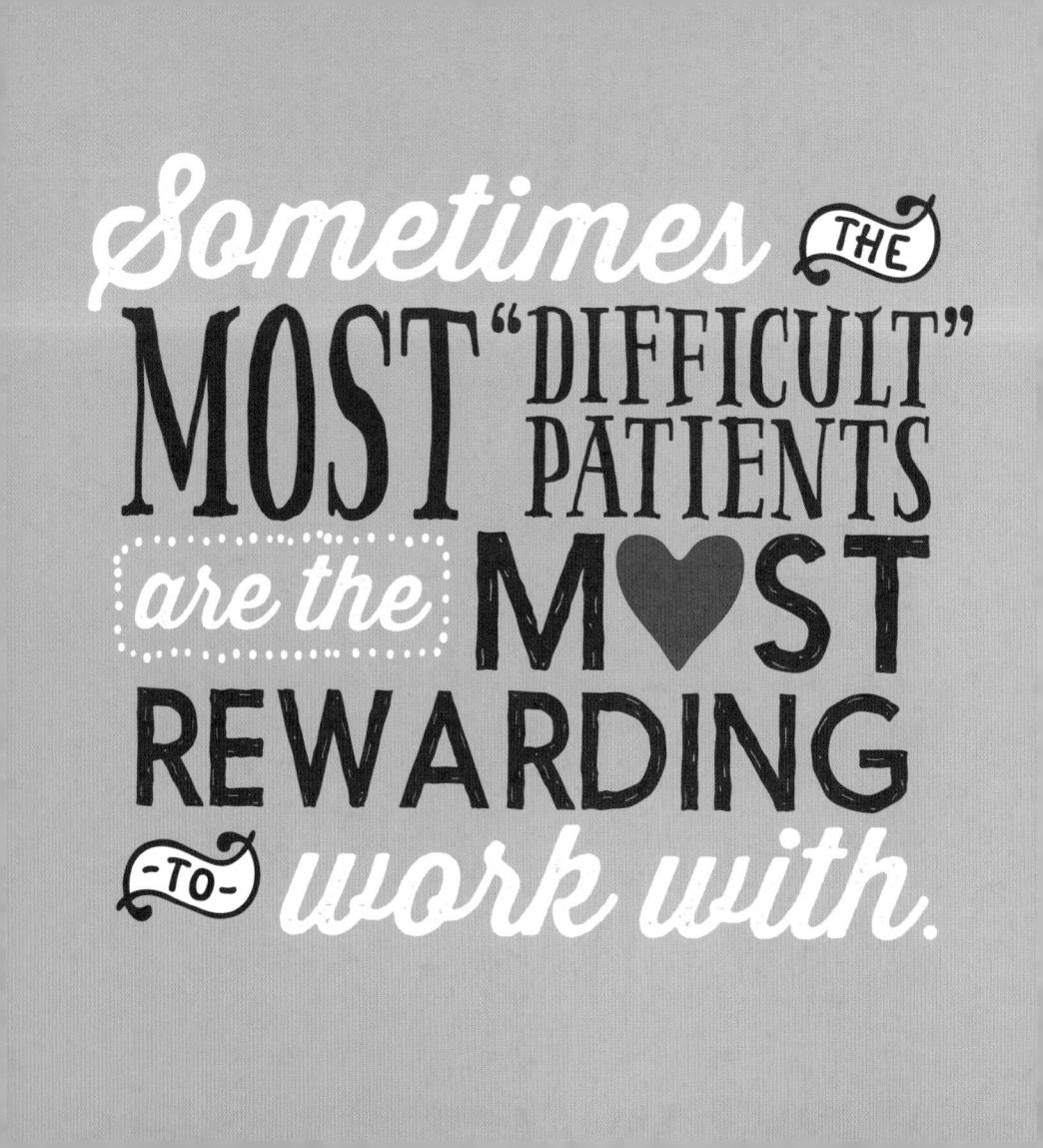
Sometimes THE
MOST "DIFFICULT" PATIENTS
are the MOST
REWARDING
-TO- work with.

You might be a nurse if...

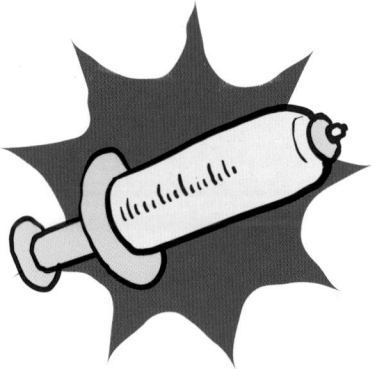

YOU KNOW THE MAGICAL POWERS OF A NORMAL SALINE FLUSH.

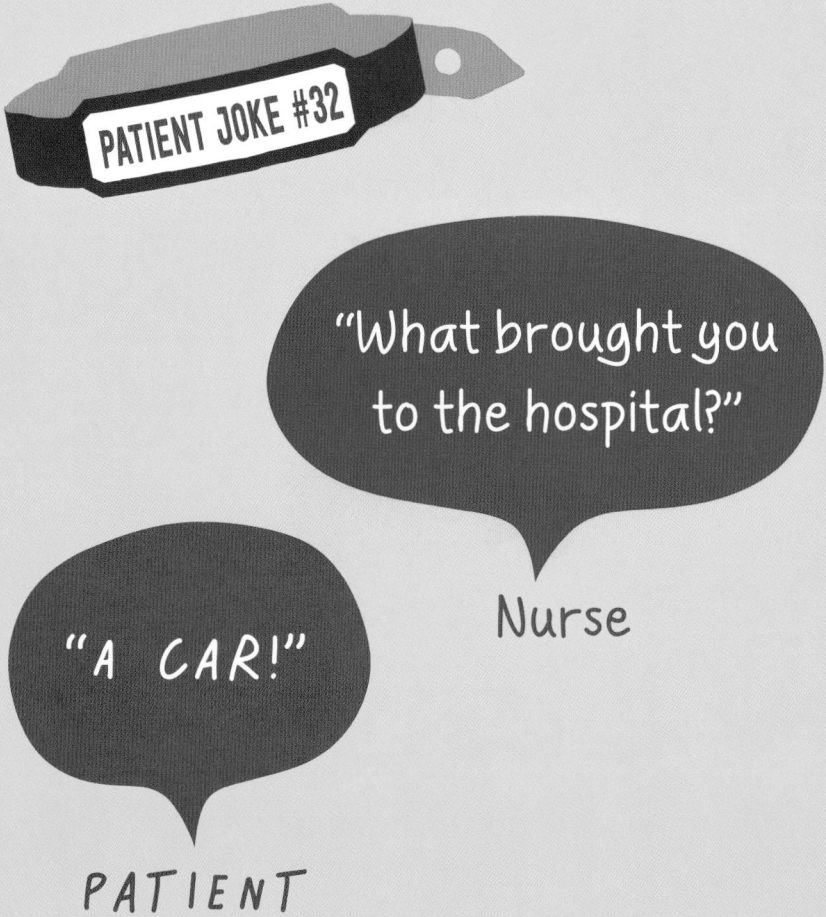
PATIENT JOKE #32
"What brought you to the hospital?"
Nurse
"A CAR!"
PATIENT

SHIFT CHANGE

might be my

ABSOLUTE FAVORITE

time of day.

Once a nurse, always a nurse.

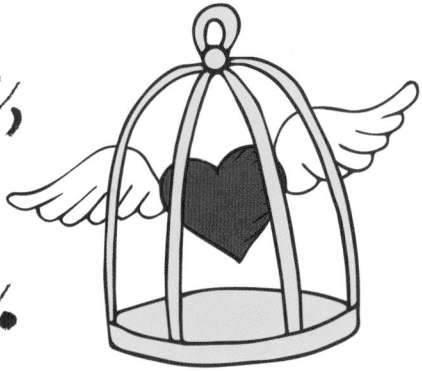

No matter where you go or what you do, you can never truly get out of nursing.

It's like the Mafia...YOU KNOW T$\overset{\frown}{\odot}\overset{\frown}{\odot}$ MUCH.

—DEB GAULDIN, RN

HOW TO MAKE A PATIENT HAPPY 101

1. Warm blankets
2. Turkey sandwiches
3. Ginger ale
4. Functioning TV
5. Repeat steps 1–4, especially 1

Always remember
your first
NURSE MENTOR
and aspire to be
like her or him.

MY BLOOD TYPE IS...

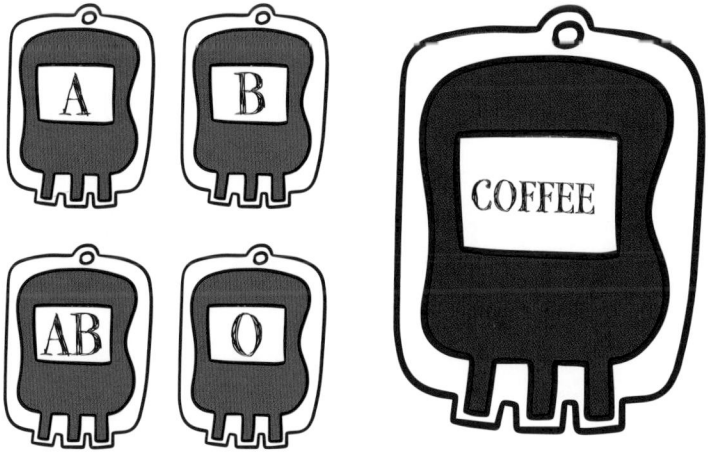

COFFEE

Which would you choose?

A

A breakroom full of delicious snacks and coffee and the ability to actually take a break!

B

All A&Ox4 independent patients.

C

A computer and mouse that are fast and fully functional.

D

Never having to wait for meds from the pharmacy.

✓ WAKE UP,

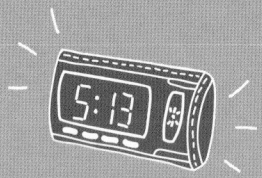

✓ THROW ON THOSE SCRUBS,

✓ FIND YOUR CAFFEINE,

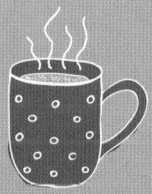

AND

✓ **BE AWESOME!**

MURPHY'S LAW OF NURSING

#47

THE POOP WILL
ALMOST ALWAYS MISS
THE CHUX PAD DESPITE
YOUR BEST EFFORTS.

YOUR BRAIN CELLS
COMING TOGETHER TO PRONOUNCE
COMPLICATED DRUG NAMES.

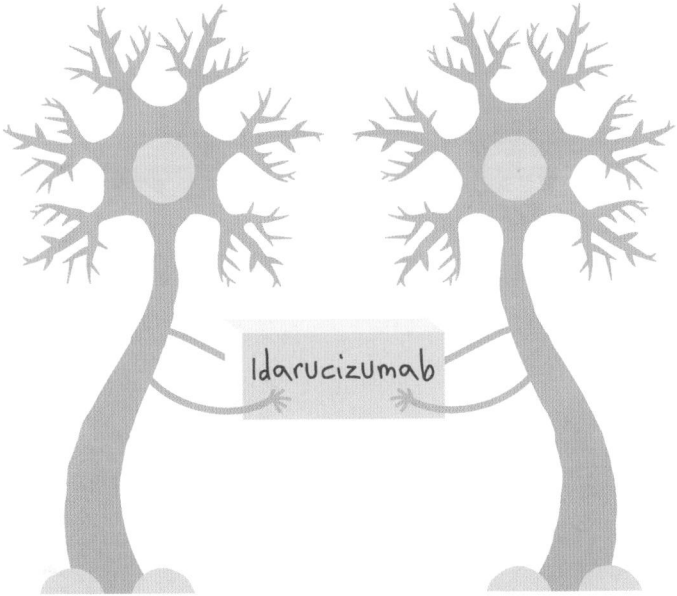

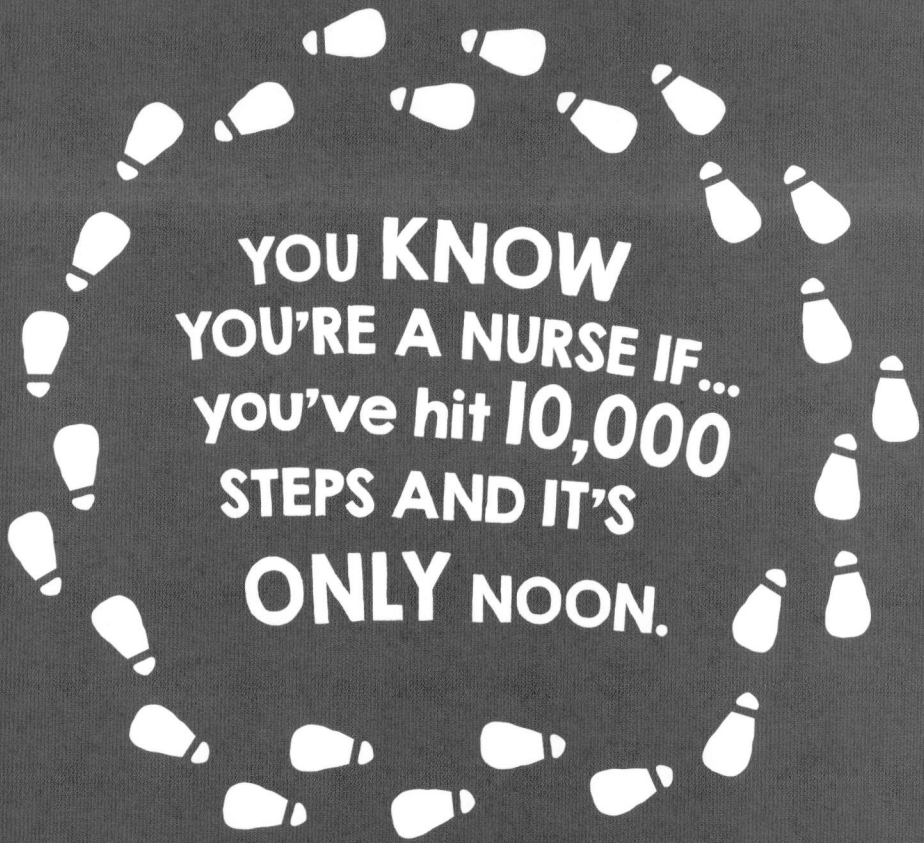
YOU KNOW
YOU'RE A NURSE IF...
you've hit 10,000
STEPS AND IT'S
ONLY NOON.

MURPHY'S LAW OF NURSING

YOU'LL FINISH YOUR CHARTING AND REALIZE YOU'RE IN THE WRONG PATIENT'S CHART.

When you finally find a tiny vein for an IV:

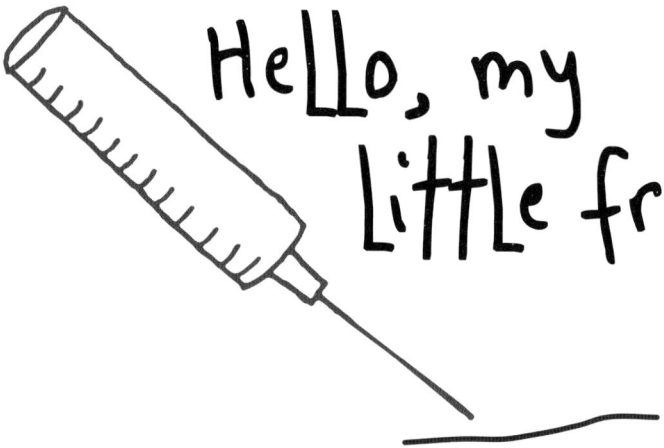

Hello, my little friend!

Nursing is a career where people from many

DIFFERENT BACKGROUNDS

come together FOR the same common goal:

to help people.

TOP SIX NURSING WANTS:

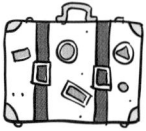

MORE VACATION.

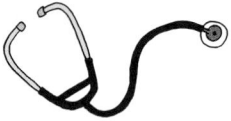

ADEQUATE STAFFING.

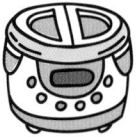

DELICIOUS POTLUCKS.

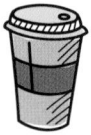

COFFEE. AT. ALL. TIMES.

KIND PATIENTS.

TO HAVE YOUR BESTIES WORKING WITH YOU EVERY SHIFT.

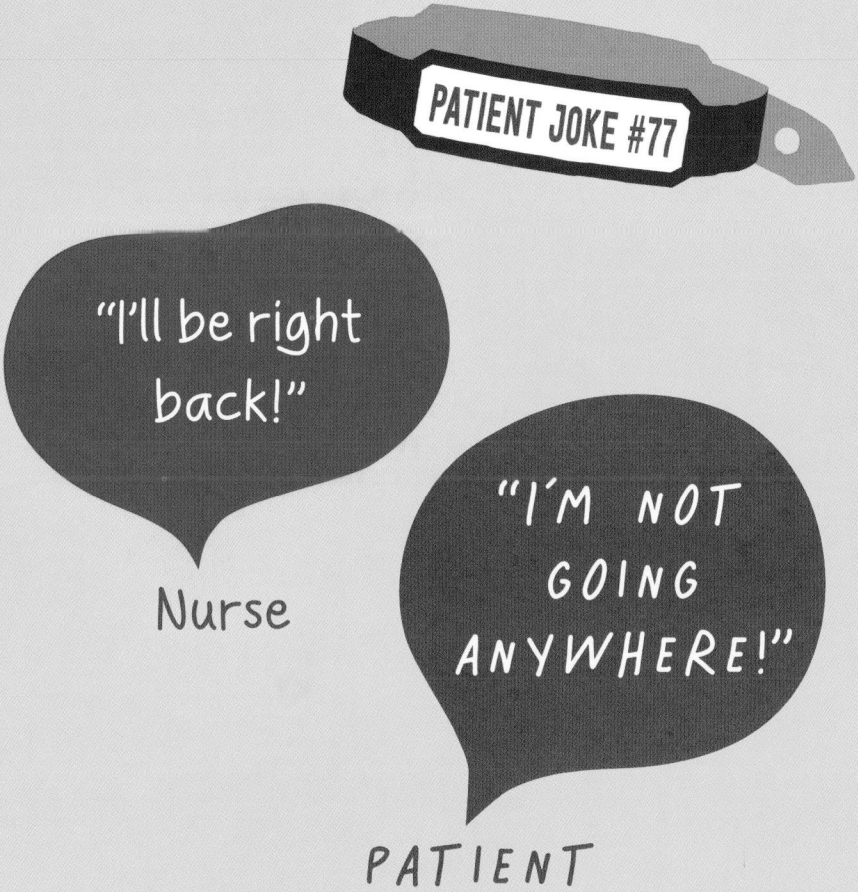
PATIENT JOKE #77
"I'll be right back!"
Nurse
"I'M NOT GOING ANYWHERE!"
PATIENT

COWORKERS
WHO HAVE A
GREAT WORK ETHIC
AND A
SENSE OF HUMOR
ARE THE BEST!

MURPHY'S LAW OF NURSING

YOU'LL GET YOUR
PATIENT SETTLED BACK
INTO BED AND THEY'LL
WANT TO GET OUT AGAIN.

There's no

innovation

like

nurse innovation

at 2 a.m. when supply doesn't have what you need and you gotta

make it work!

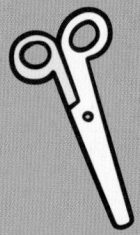

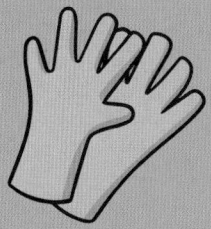

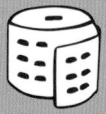

There are 4 types of people during a CODE BLUE– which are you?

1. YASSS! GET ME IN THERE!
2. I'll take care of the other patients!
3. Wait, there was a code blue?
4. ANYONE NEED A GLUCOMETER?

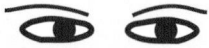

Nursing pet peeve #7:

Tattoos, shirts, stickers...

OKAY, BASICALLY

anything

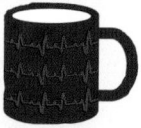

WITH AN EKG RHYTHM

that doesn't actually look

like a real rhythm.

America's nurses

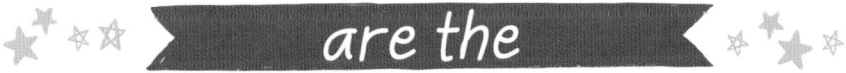

beating heart

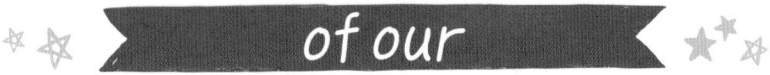

MEDICAL SYSTEM.

—BARACK OBAMA,
44TH PRESIDENT OF THE UNITED STATES

NURSES ARE THERE WHEN the last breath is taken, AND NURSES ARE THERE WHEN the first breath is taken. ALTHOUGH IT IS MORE ENJOYABLE to celebrate the birth, IT IS JUST AS IMPORTANT to comfort in death.

—Christine Bell, author

TINY BLESSINGS #19

When your patient's electrolyte labs come back within normal range and you don't have to replace them!

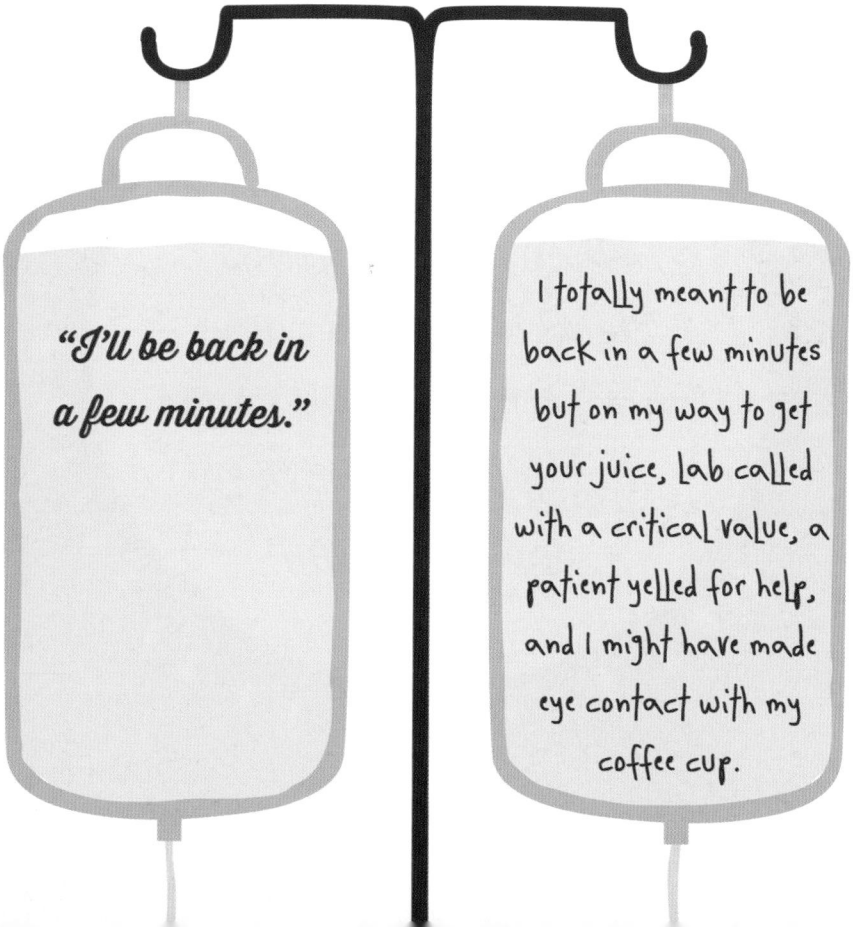
WHAT I SAID:
WHAT IT ACTUALLY MEANS:
"I'll be back in a few minutes."
I totally meant to be back in a few minutes but on my way to get your juice, lab called with a critical value, a patient yelled for help, and I might have made eye contact with my coffee cup.

DOCTOR'S ORDERS THAT MAKE YOU GROAN

#7

Give 120mg furosemide

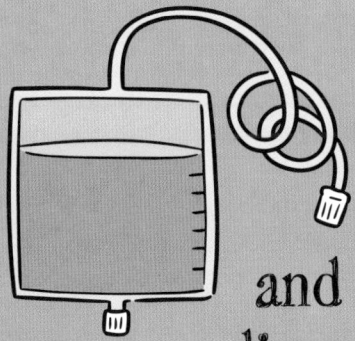

and discontinue catheter.

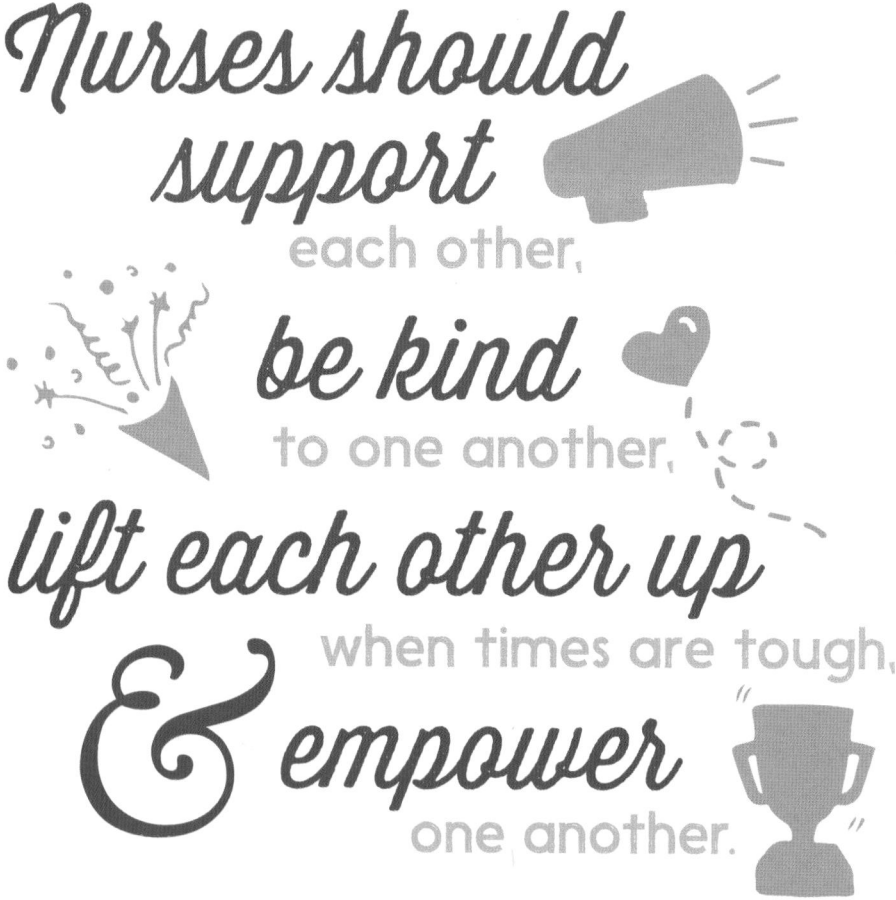
Nurses should support
each other,
be kind
to one another,
lift each other up
when times are tough,
& empower
one another.

WORK ALL DAY: EAT NOTHING.

GET OFF WORK: INHALE BOAT-LOAD OF CARBS BEFORE FALLING ASLEEP 15 MINUTES LATER.

The bladder scanner,
pill crusher,
and EKG machine:

ALL HARDER TO FIND THAN WALDO.

Nurses

—one of the few *blessings* of being ill.

—Sara Moss-Wolfe, occupation unknown

TWO POSITIVES TO CRYING IN THE BATHROOM DURING AN OVERWHELMING DAY:

- ☑ YOU'RE GETTING A LITTLE BREAK.
- ☑ TECHNICALLY YOU'RE BEING PAID TO CRY.

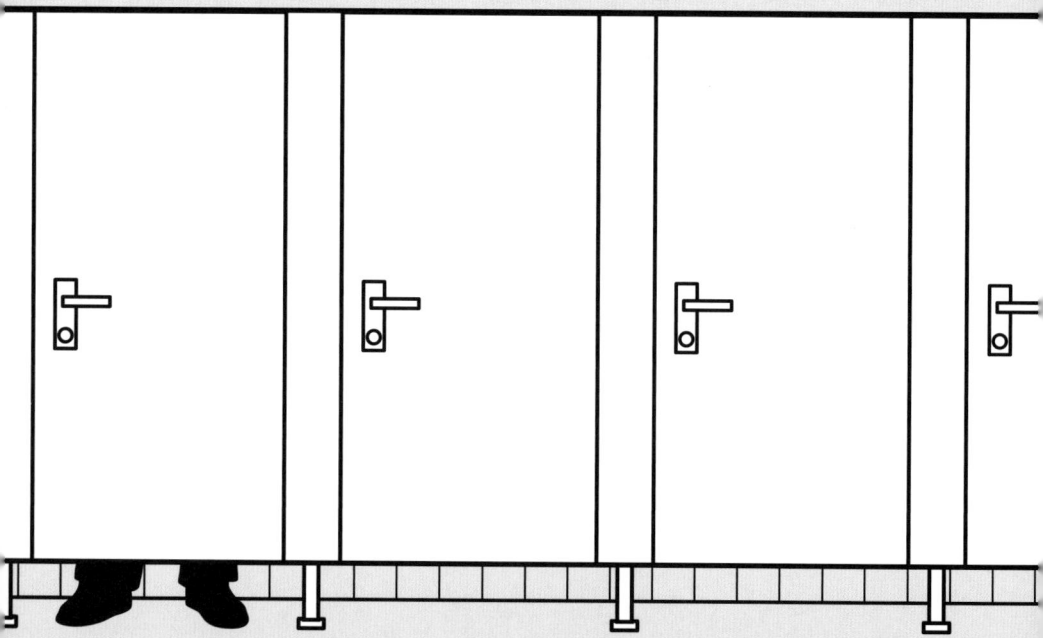

There's no satisfaction

like when the INTERN says

but the ATTENDING says

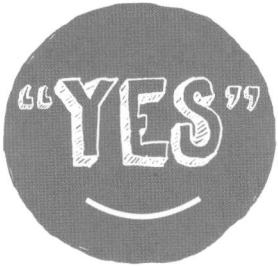

You know you're a nurse if...

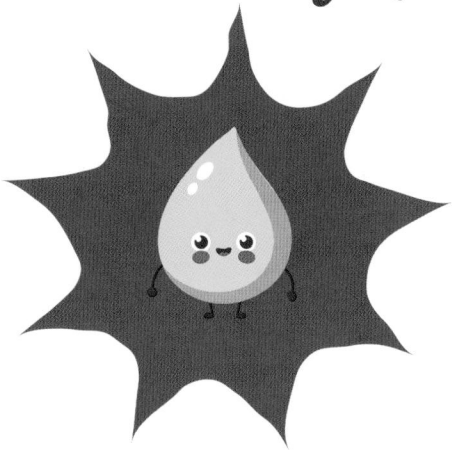

YOU FEEL A LIQUID LAND ON YOUR SHOE AND SOAK INTO YOUR SOCK AND YOU HOPE IT'S JUST URINE.

I'M SORRY TO SAY,
BUT WE ARE PROBABLY
GOING TO HAVE TO
DRAW SOME BLOOD.

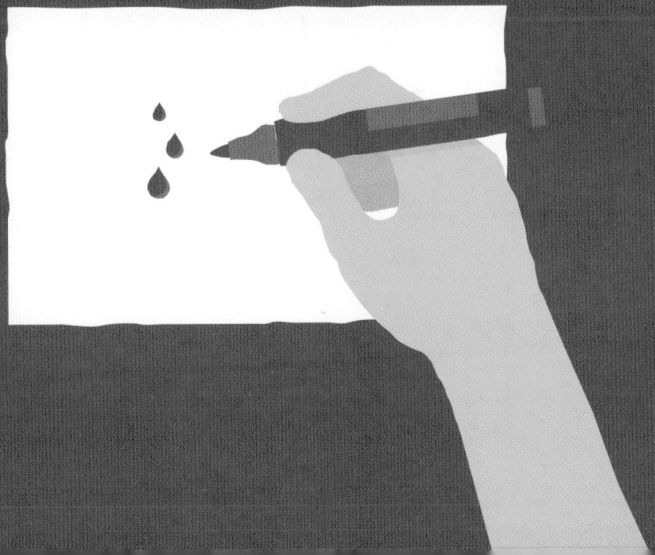

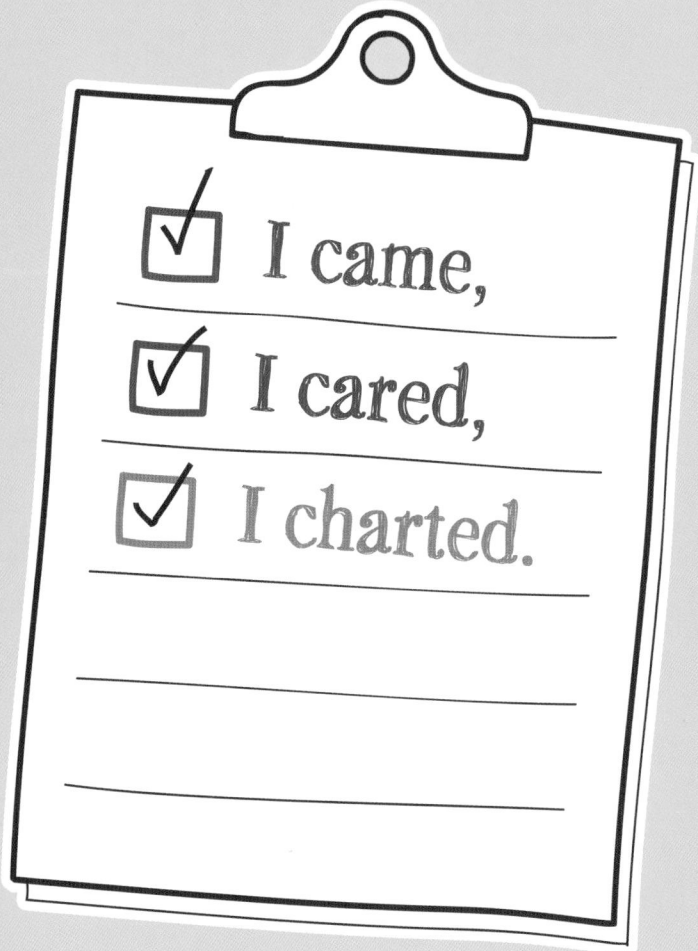
I came,
I cared,
I charted.

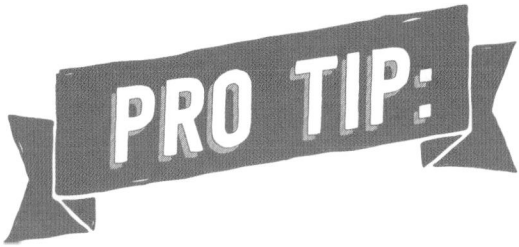

You can't get an admission if no one can find you!

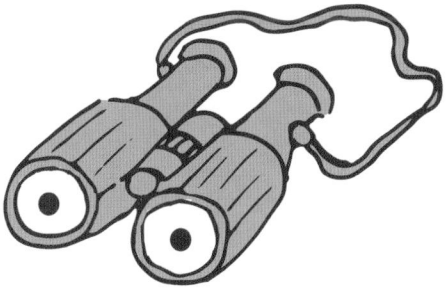

JUUUUUST KIDDING!

TINY BLESSINGS #57

When your patient's blood sugar is just below the level to give sliding scale insulin!

STRANGE THINGS NURSES FIND THEMSELVES SAYING:

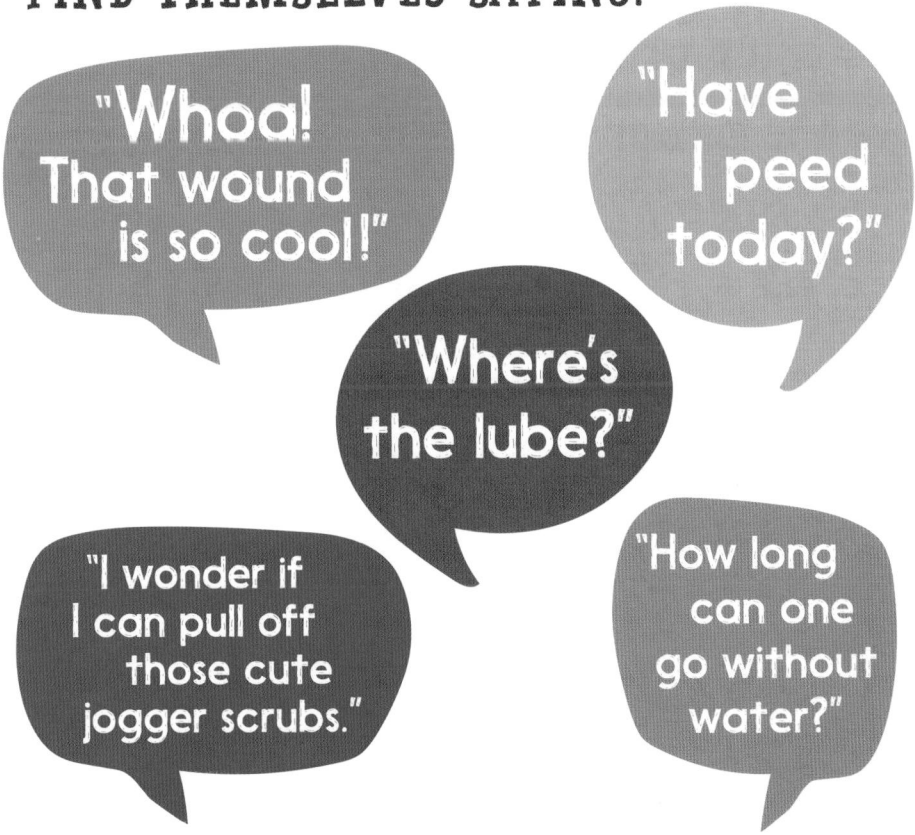

Too often we underestimate the power of a *touch*, a *smile*, a *kind word*, a *listening ear*, an *honest accomplishment*, or the *smallest act of caring*, all of which have the potential to *turn a life around*.

—Leo Buscaglia, author

WHENEVER I HEAR A PERSON SAY

someone made their heart

SKIP A BEAT,

all I can think is

THAT'S AN ARRHYTHMIA

and probably should be

CHECKED OUT.

THERE'S NO ANXIETY LIKE THE ANXIETY OF GOING BACK TO WORK AFTER TWO WEEKS OF VACATION.

WILL I REMEMBER MY PASSWORDS?

DO I KNOW HOW TO DO MY JOB STILL?

WILL I GET THE HARDEST ASSIGNMENT?

WHAT IF MY ALARM DOESN'T GO OFF?

MURPHY'S LAW OF NURSING

EVERY TIME THE HOSPITAL
BUYS NEW PATIENT BEDS,
THE FITTED SHEETS
WILL BE TOO SMALL.

NURSE FACT:

IT'S YOUR NIGHT OFF *and the only clothes you know fit are* SCRUBS & YOGA PANTS.

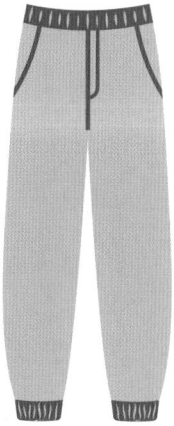

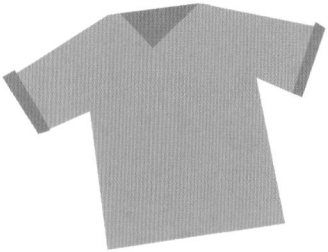

MY ATTEMPT AT GENERIC DRUG NAMES:

jalkwjfoaweutoawutoatwuoptjdsfmab

SOMETIMES

I want someone to hug me and say,

"I KNOW THIS SHIFT HAS BEEN ROUGH, BUT IT'S GOING TO BE OKAY. HERE'S SOME CHOCOLATE, COFFEE, A THERAPY DOG TO PET, AND $1.5 MILLION."

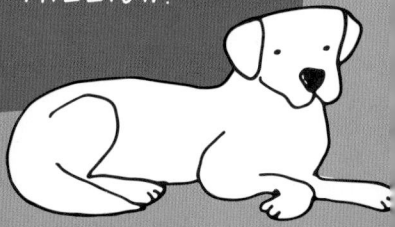

WHAT MAKES YOU THE HAPPIEST?

YOU CAN ONLY PICK ONE!

Getting a lunch break

Having your patient be adorable and thankful

Therapy dogs visiting

When your patient uses their incentive spirometer without prompting

When patients take meds via med cup instead of their hands

THERE'S NO
CARDIO
LIKE CHEST
COMPRESSION
CARDIO.

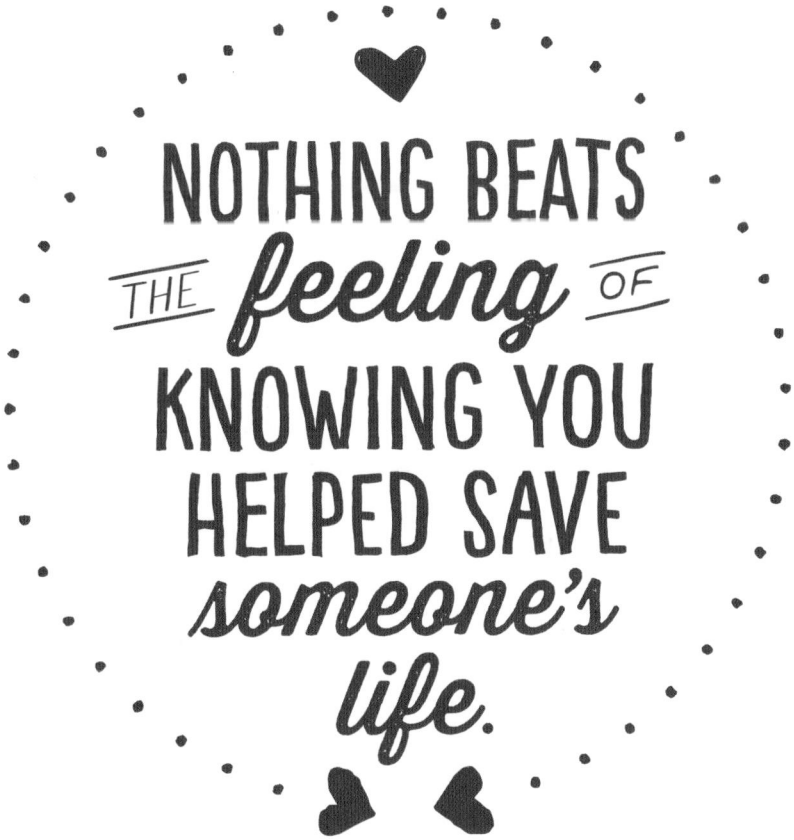
NOTHING BEATS
THE feeling OF
KNOWING YOU
HELPED SAVE
someone's
life.

When in doubt,
just take a deep breath.
Inhale the good stuff,
exhale the bad stuff.

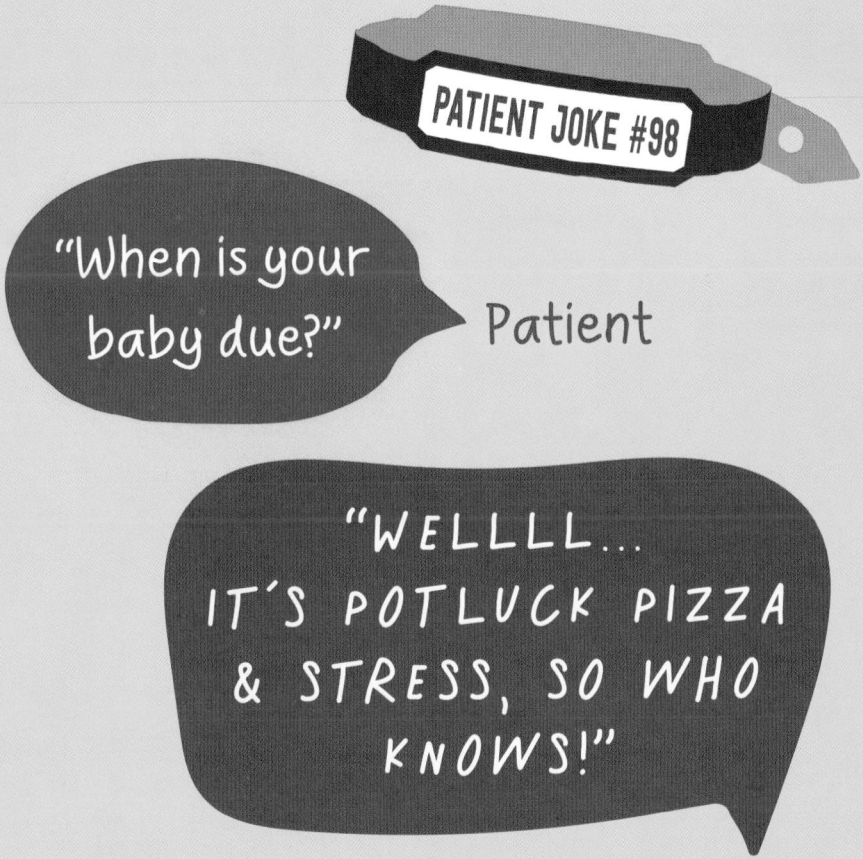
PATIENT JOKE #98
"When is your baby due?"
Patient
"WELLLL... IT'S POTLUCK PIZZA & STRESS, SO WHO KNOWS!"
NURSE

ME AS A NEW NURSE:

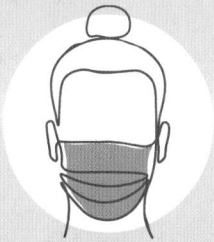

Fifteen Minutes Early for Shift

New Pens in Pocket

Pristine Scrubs in a Fun Pattern

Hair in Cute Topknot

Shiny Clean Stethoscope

ME FIVE YEARS IN:

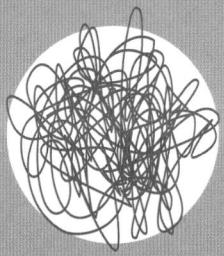

Barely On Time for Shift

No Pen

OR Scrubs from Some Other Hospital

Hair Sprayed with Dry Shampoo

Where's My Stethoscope?

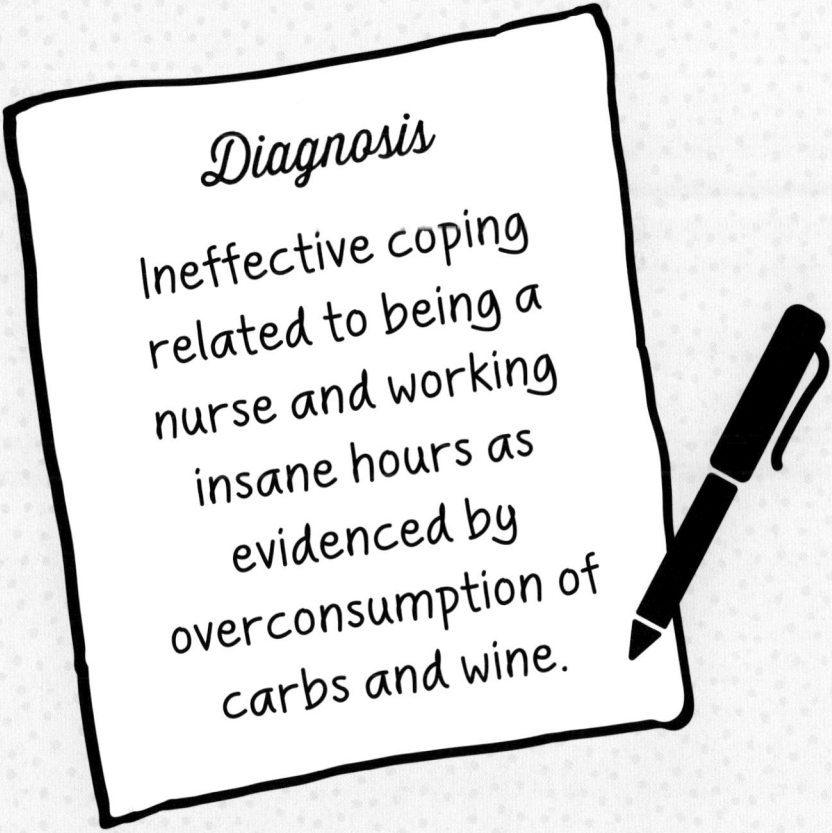
Diagnosis
Ineffective coping related to being a nurse and working insane hours as evidenced by overconsumption of carbs and wine.

Nursing:

You just have to take it one

"you've got to be kidding me"

at a time.

BE *teachable.*

BE *humble.*

BE *a team player.*

BE THE TYPE OF NURSE YOU WANT TO WORK WITH.

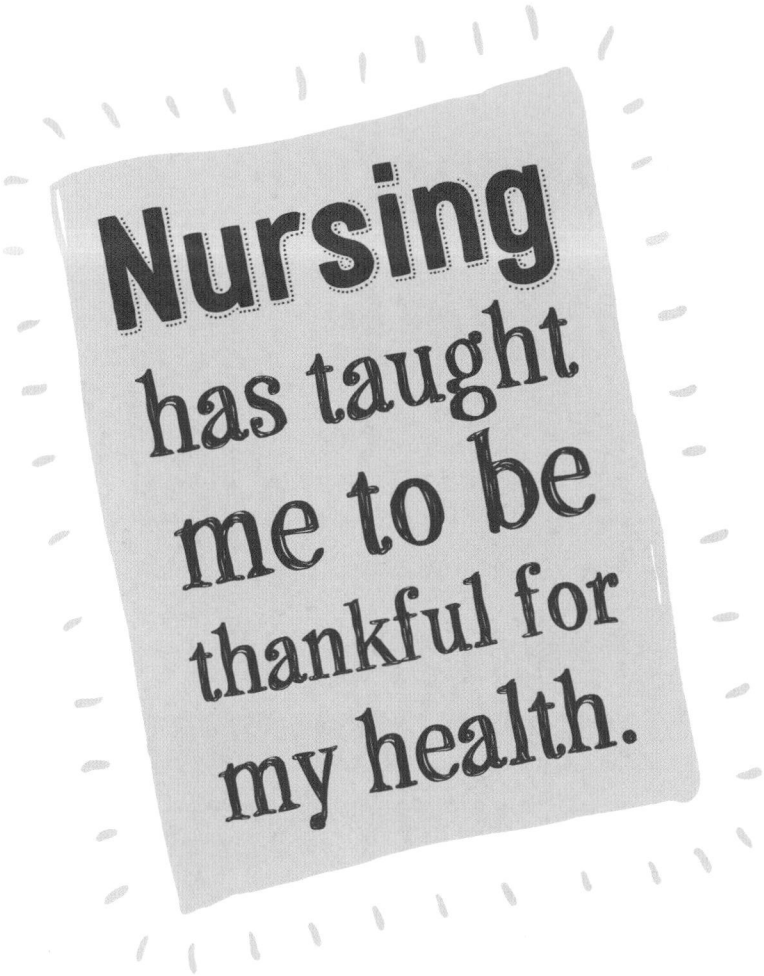
Nursing
has taught
me to be
thankful for
my health.

TINY BLESSINGS #77

When a call light rings and the patient says it was an accident!

NURSING GOLD MEDAL

WHEN YOUR PATIENT SAYS THEY'RE A DIFFICULT STICK AND YOU SEE THAT FLASH OF BLOOD RETURN!

You have not lived today

UNTIL YOU HAVE

done something

FOR *someone*

who can never repay you.

—JOHN BUNYAN,
AUTHOR AND PURITAN PREACHER

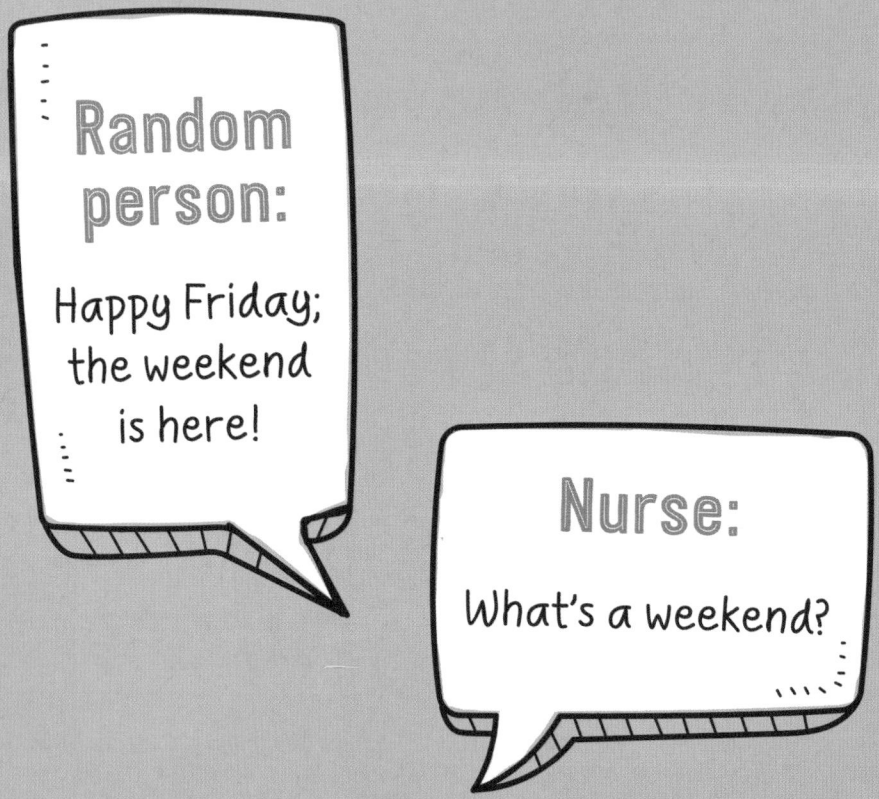
Random person:
Happy Friday; the weekend is here!
Nurse:
What's a weekend?

Are you even a nurse
if you don't think

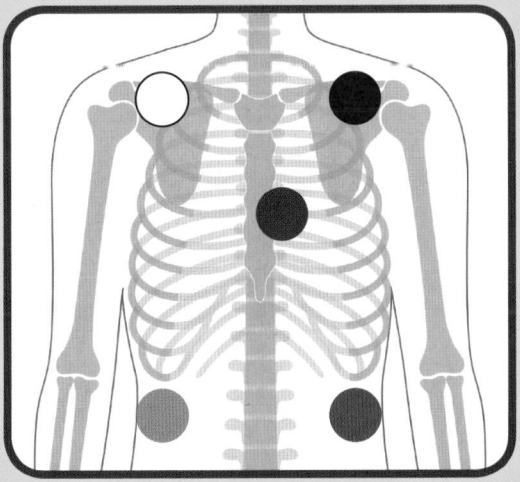

"SMOKE OVER FIRE"

while putting on EKG leads?

APPLYING TED HOSE
IS LIKE TRYING TO
SQUEEZE
A
WATERMELON
INTO SOCKS.

BETWEEN 3–4 A.M. ON THE NIGHT SHIFT:

WHEN EVERYTHING IS FUNNY

Night Shift Nurses' WORST ENEMIES

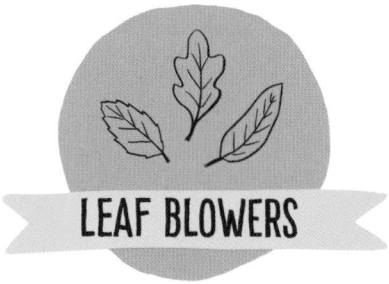

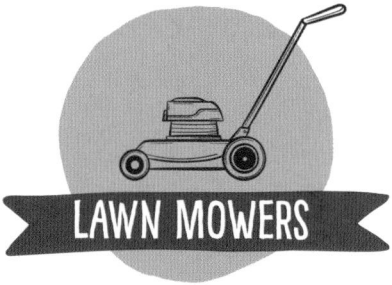

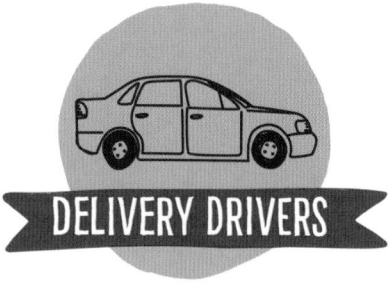

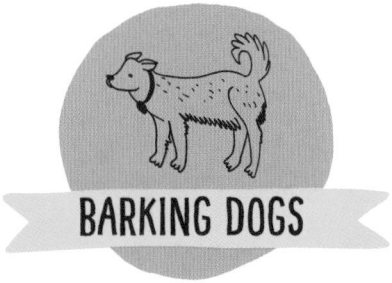

WHEN SOMEONE
is going
through a storm,
your silent presence
IS MORE POWERFUL
than a million
empty words.

—MAHATMA GANDHI, LAWYER,
POLITICIAN, AND SOCIAL ACTIVIST

MURPHY'S LAW OF NURSING

YOU PAGE THE DOC FOR SOMETHING SUPER IMPORTANT AND WHEN THEY CALL BACK, YOU CAN'T REMEMBER THE PATIENT'S NAME.

DO NO HARM,
take NO
NONSENSE.

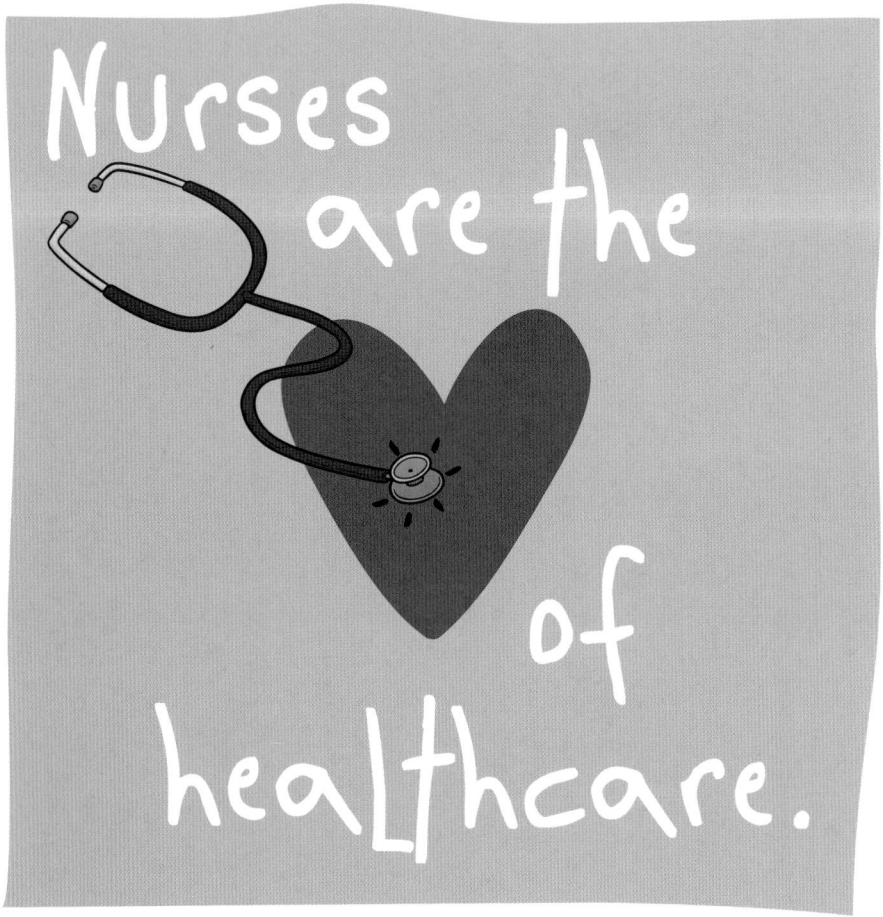
Nurses
are the
of
healthcare.

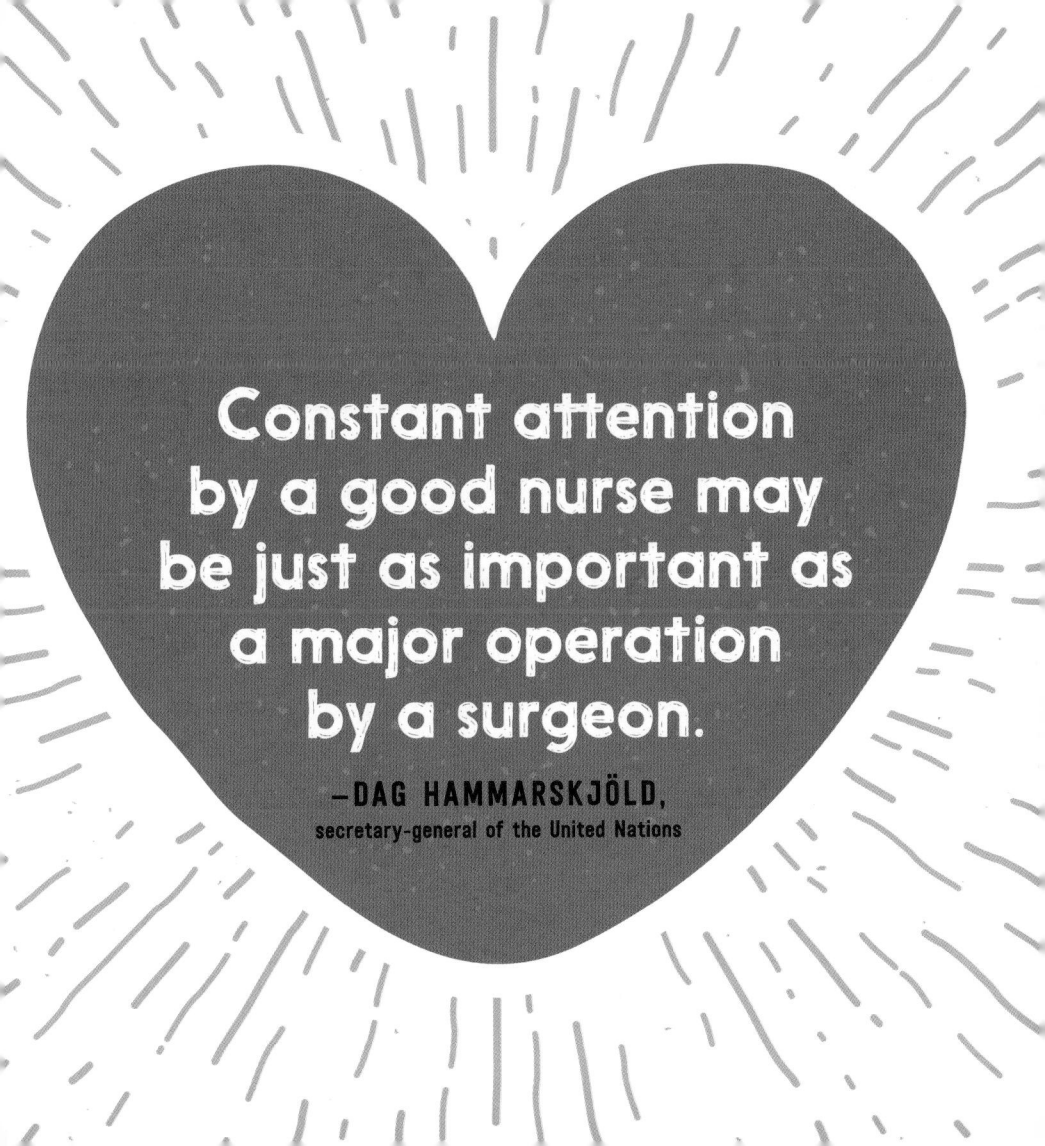
Constant attention by a good nurse may be just as important as a major operation by a surgeon.
—DAG HAMMARSKJÖLD,
secretary-general of the United Nations

You know you're a nurse if...

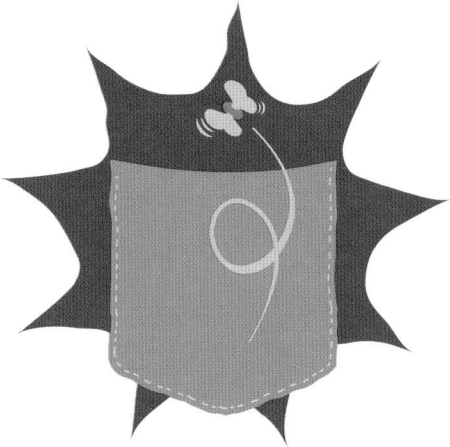

YOU'RE DIGGING IN YOUR POCKETS FOR CASH TO GET A SNACK AND ONLY COME OUT WITH CRUMPLED ALCOHOL SWABS AND A HEPARIN SHOT YOUR PATIENT REFUSED.

DOCTOR'S ORDERS THAT MAKE YOU GROAN

#88

Insert nasogastric tube

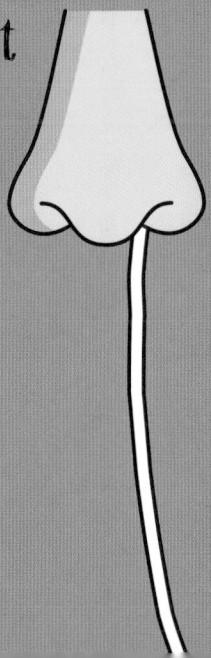

on your awake patient.

WHAT I SAID:

WHAT I DID:

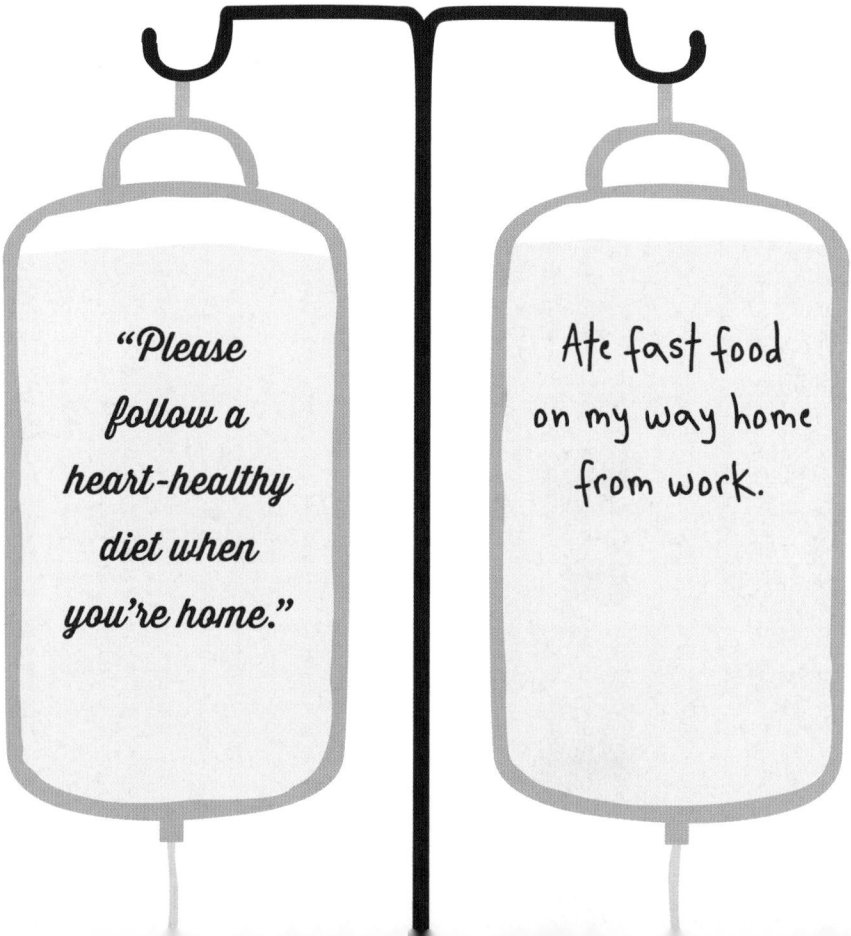

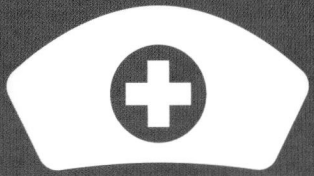

KEEP
CALM
AND
CHART
ON

Aspire to be
THAT ONE OG NURSE
WHO KNOWS HER STUFF
AND TELLS EVERYONE
WHAT SHE THINKS
without reservation.

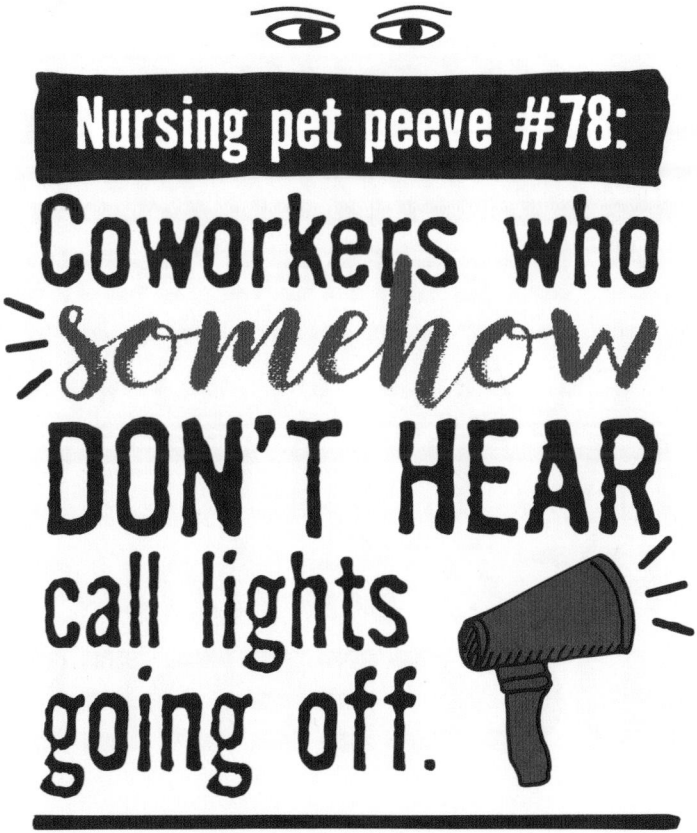
Nursing pet peeve #78:
Coworkers who
somehow
DON'T HEAR
call lights
going off.

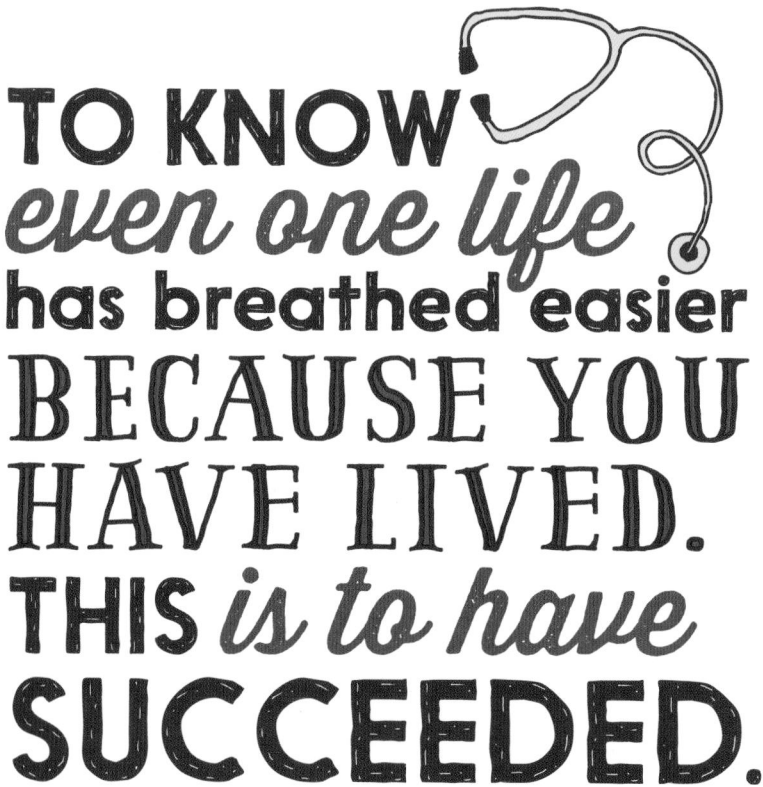

—Ralph Waldo Emerson, poet

A Poem about Work:

Coffee Coffee,
Meds/Walks/Alarms,
Drive home,
Wine.

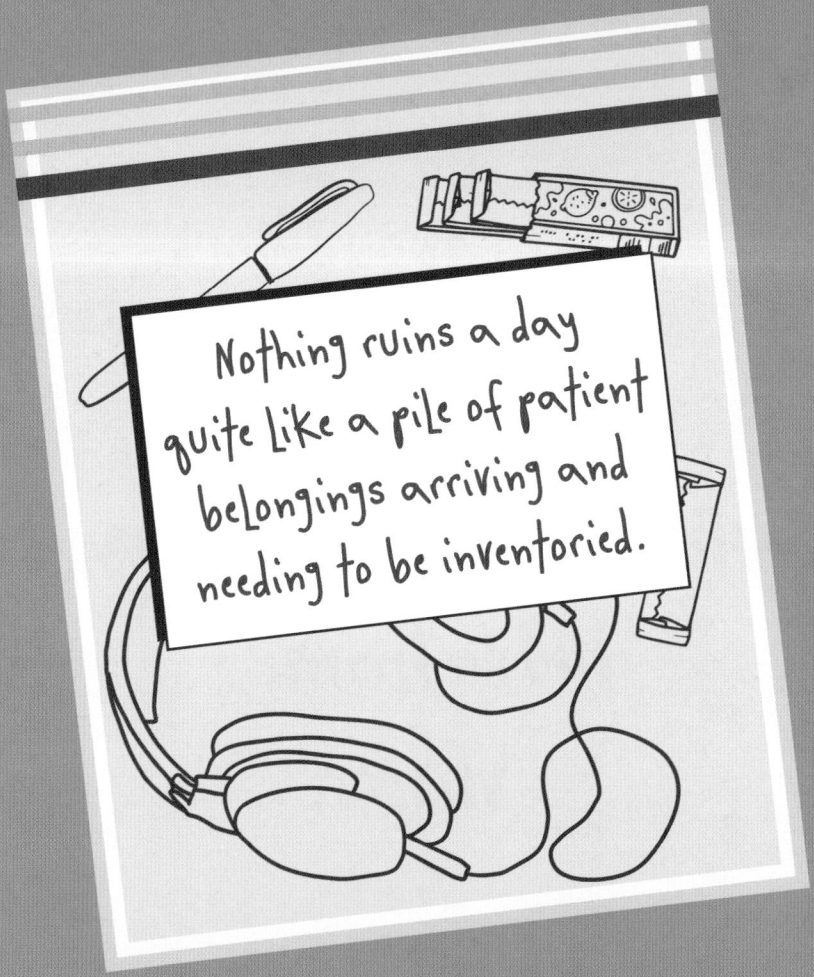
Nothing ruins a day quite like a pile of patient belongings arriving and needing to be inventoried.

Three questions that make a nurse's eyes roll:

ARE YOU GOING TO MARRY A DOCTOR?

WHY DIDN'T YOU BECOME A DOCTOR?

WHY ARE YOU SO TIRED, YOU ONLY WORK THREE DAYS A WEEK?

You know you're getting

HANGRY

when your patient's

meal tray starts to look

appetizing.

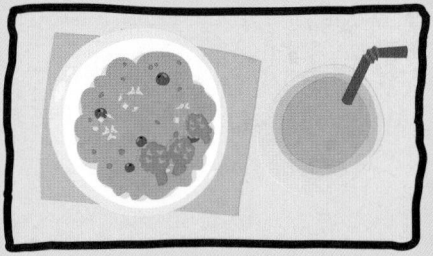

LET US NEVER CONSIDER OURSELVES FINISHED NURSES.

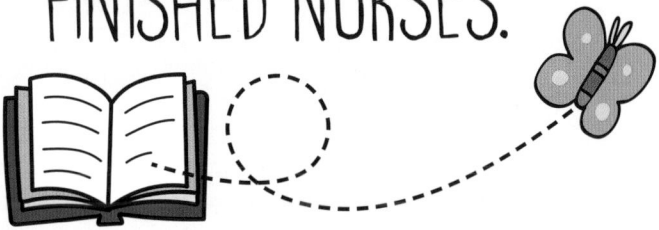

WE MUST BE LEARNING ALL OF OUR LIVES.

–Florence Nightingale,
founder of modern nursing

I'm thankful for:

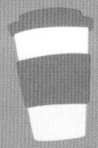

coffee

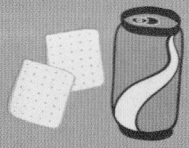

nutrition room snacks

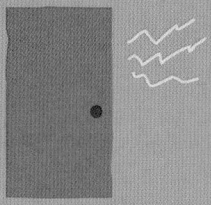

the med room where I can vent to my coworker

patients who use their call light sparingly

TINY BLESSINGS #99

When your patient's ID band and IV are above the covers and you can scan and hook up their IV without waking them!

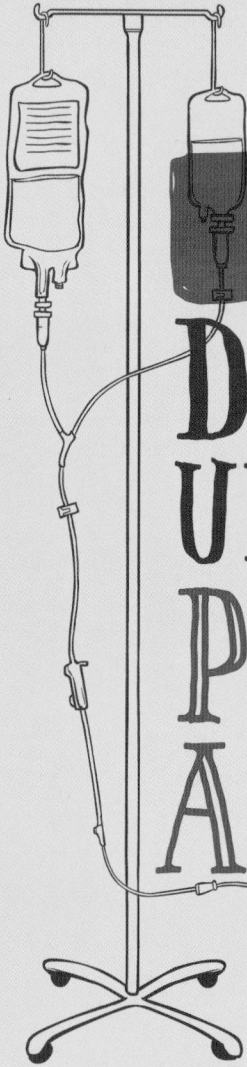

Psssst!

DID YOU UNCLAMP YOUR PIGGYBACK ANTIBIOTIC?

You know you're a nurse if...

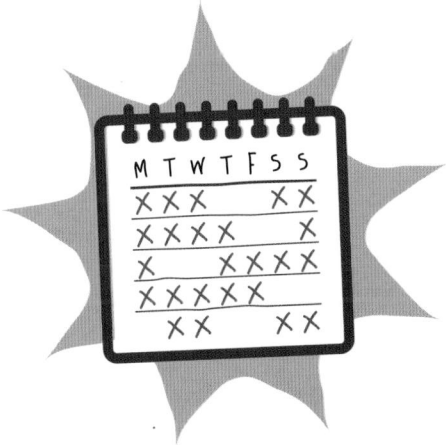

YOU'VE EXPLAINED YOUR SCHEDULE TO YOUR FAMILY A MILLION TIMES AND THEY STILL ASK YOU TO DO THINGS ON THE DAYS YOU WORK.

I think a

hero

is any person really intent on making this a better place for all people.

—Maya Angelou, poet

Lessons from Patients

IF THIS LITTLE PIGGY STARTS LOOKING A LITTLE STRANGE, COME IN RIGHT AWAY!

HOW CAN ANYBODY HATE NURSES?

NOBODY HATES NURSES.

The only time you hate a nurse is when they're giving you an enema.

—Warren Beatty, actor

Every morning,

make sure to take a moment to think of all the things you're GRATEFUL for...

BEFORE HEADING INTO WORK
AND BEING ANNOYED
ABOUT EVERY LITTLE THING.

You know you're a nurse if...

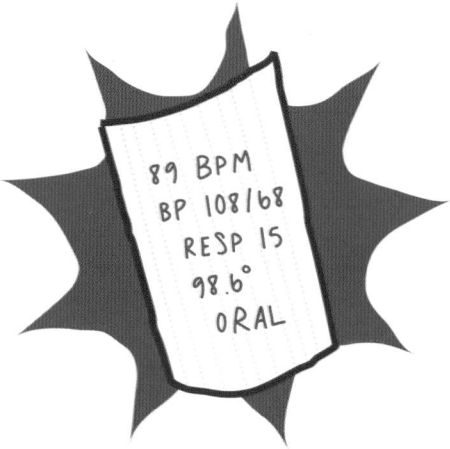

YOU USE A PAPER TOWEL TO WRITE DOWN VITAL SIGNS.

LIVE LIFE WHEN YOU HAVE IT.

Life

is a splendid gift—

there is nothing small about it.

—FLORENCE NIGHTINGALE, FOUNDER OF MODERN NURSING

LIFE'S MOST PERSISTENT and URGENT QUESTION IS,

"WHAT ARE YOU DOING FOR OTHERS?"

—Martin Luther King Jr., minister, activist, and civil rights leader

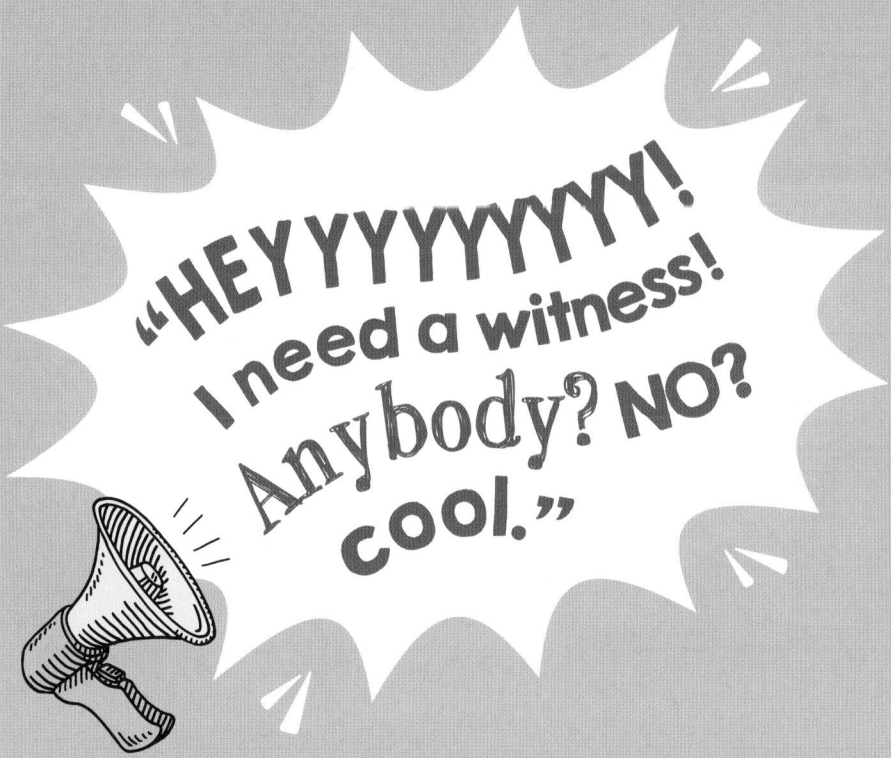
"HEYYYYYYYY!
I need a witness!
Anybody? NO?
cool."

It's important to realize EACH DAY THAT A PATIENT IS PUTTING THEIR LIFE IN YOUR HANDS & *what a privilege that is.*

IT'S OKAY *to cry*
after a REALLY TOUGH SHIFT.
VULNERABILITY AND
SORTING THROUGH *your* FEELINGS
is part of
SELF-CARE.

DOCTOR'S ORDERS THAT MAKE YOU GROAN

#101

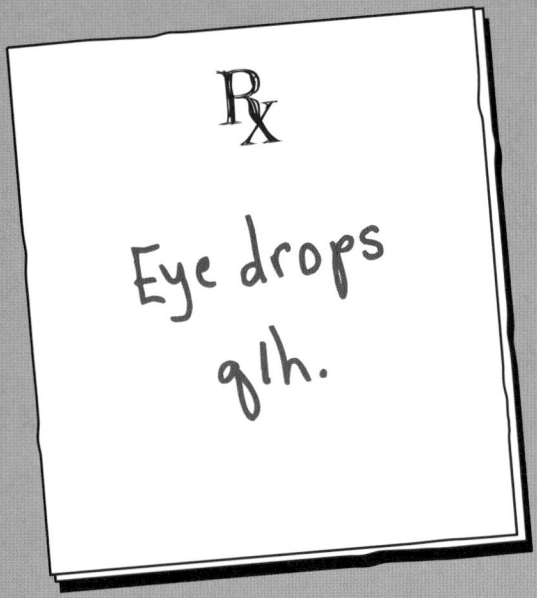

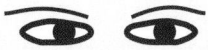

Nursing pet peeve #98:

NURSE: I have a missing antibiotic, can you send it up?

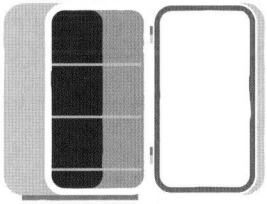

PHARMACY: Have you checked the fridge?

TINY BLESSINGS #157

When you catch your IV infusion before it runs dry.

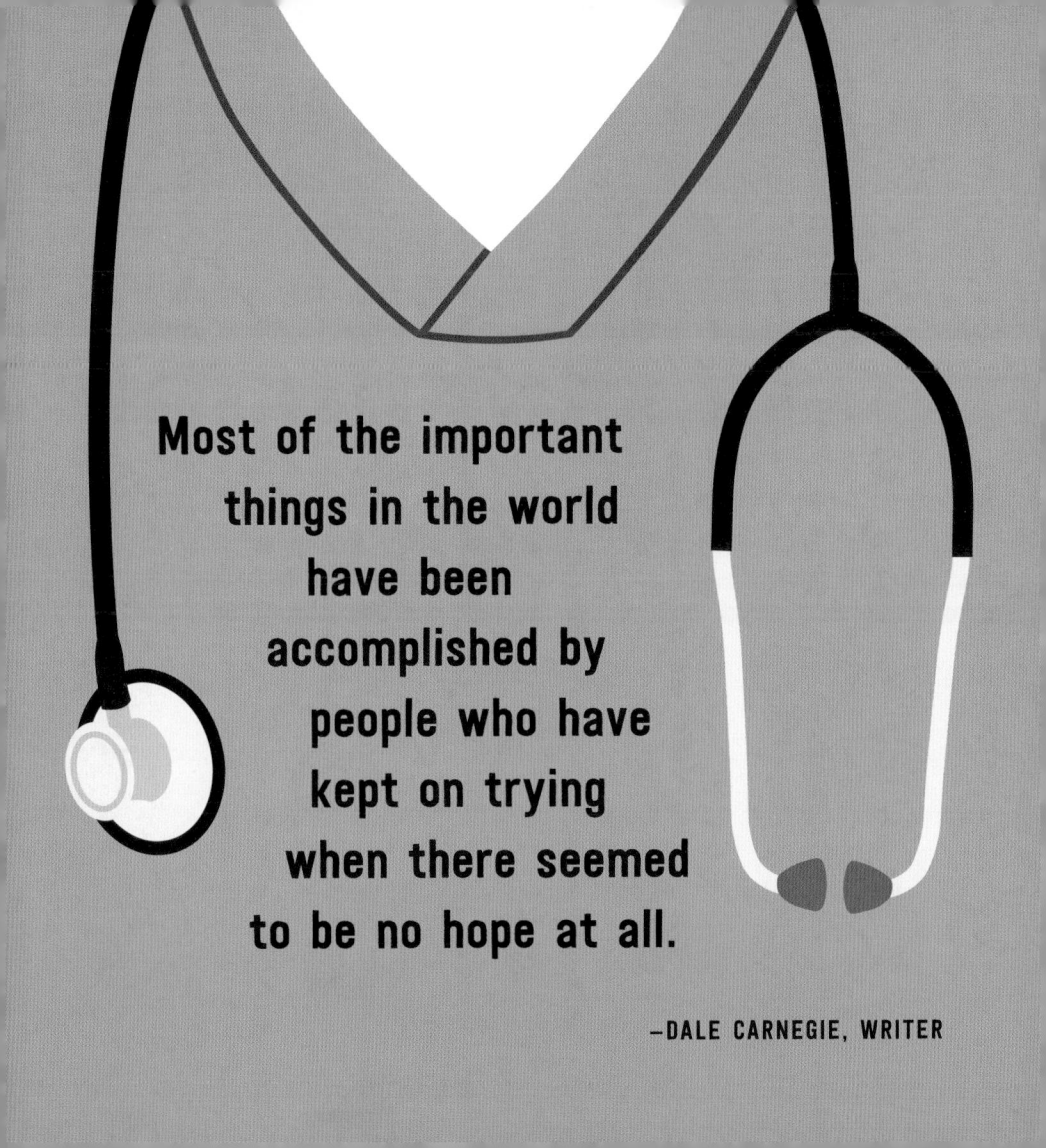
Most of the important things in the world have been accomplished by people who have kept on trying when there seemed to be no hope at all.
–DALE CARNEGIE, WRITER

YES!

I charted that I charted what I previously charted.

WAIT, HOLD ON!

I have to chart that I told you about my charting.

—AUTHOR UNKNOWN

WHAT *I love* MOST ABOUT NURSING

(SELECT ALL THAT APPLY):

- ☑ **Helping people to hopefully get back to their baseline**
- ☑ **A fast-paced learning environment**
- ☑ **Seeing the advancement of the medical world**
- ☑ **My coworkers**
- ☑ **Eating the patient snacks**

WHEN THE SHIFTS GET TOUGH,

remember why you became a nurse.

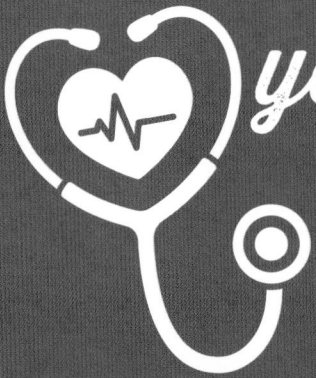

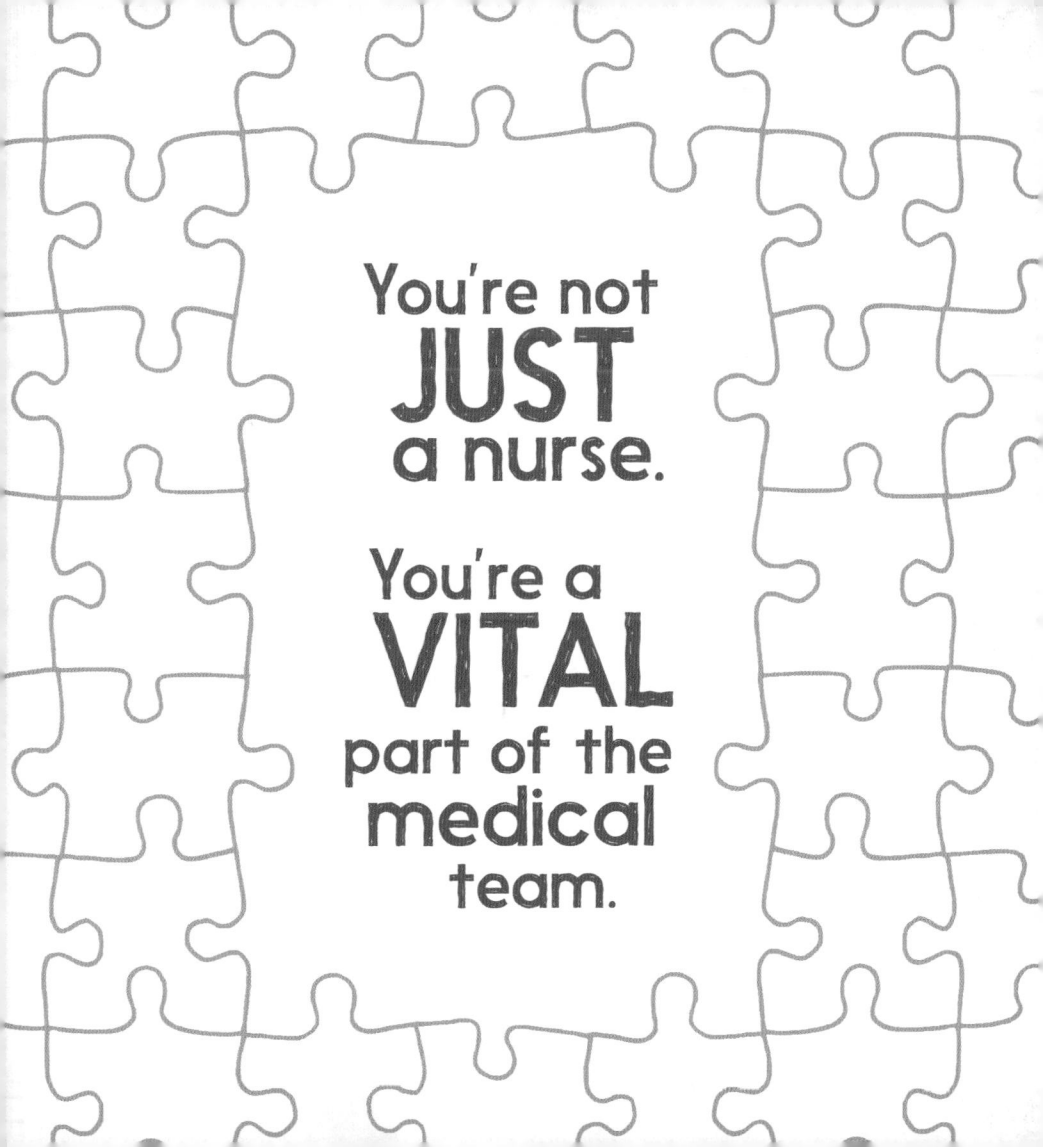
You're not
JUST
a nurse.
You're a
VITAL
part of the
medical
team.

About the Author

snarkynurses is an online community of healthcare professionals created by a critical care nurse who absolutely loves to make people laugh! From CNA to RN, med-surg to critical care, she has spent more than twelve years in the medical profession. She loves her career at the bedside but credits humor and networking with peers for keeping her sane.